OBSTETRIC
and GYNECOLOGIC
PHYSICAL THERAPY

CLINICS IN PHYSICAL THERAPY
VOLUME 20

Already Published

OBSTETRIC and GYNECOLOGIC PHYSICAL THERAPY

Edited by

Elaine Wilder, R.P.T., M.A.C.T.

Clinical Assistant Professor
Division of Physical Therapy
Department of Rehabilitation Medicine
Emory University School of Medicine
Atlanta, Georgia

CHURCHILL LIVINGSTONE
NEW YORK, EDINBURGH, LONDON, MELBOURNE
1988

Library of Congress Cataloging-in-Publication Data

Obstetric and gynecologic physical therapy.

  (Clinics in physical therapy ; v. 20)
  Includes bibliographies and index.
  1. Physical therapy. 2. Gynecology. 3. Obstetrics.
I. Wilder, Elaine. II. Series. [DNLM: 1. Gynecology.
2. Obstetrics. 3. Physical Therapy. W1 CL831CN v.20 /
WQ 100 0132]
RG129.P45027 1988   618   88-18950
ISBN 0-443-08545-5

© **Churchill Livingstone Inc. 1988**

Distributed in the United Kingdom by Churchill Livingstone, Robert Stevenson House, 1-3 Baxter's Place, Leith Walk, Edinburgh EH1 3AF, and by associated companies, branches, and representatives throughout the world.

Accurate indications, adverse reactions, and dosage schedules for drugs are provided in this book, but it is possible that they may change. The reader is urged to review the package information data of the manufacturers of the medications mentioned.

The Publishers have made every effort to trace the copyright holders for borrowed material. If they have inadvertently overlooked any, they will be pleased to make the necessary arrangements at the first opportunity.

Acquisitions Editor: *Kim Loretucci*
Copy Editor: *David Terry*
Production Designer: *Angela Cirnigliaro*
Production Supervisor: *Jocelyn Eckstein*

Printed in the United States of America

First published in 1988

To Brittany,
whose conception, gestation,
and birth paralleled the development of this project,
and to Robert,
who has given his continuous support

Contributors

Jill Schiff Boissonnault, M.S., P.T.
Physical Therapist, Physical Therapy Orthopaedic Specialists, Inc., Minneapolis, Minnesota

William G. Boissonnault, M.S., P.T.
Physical Therapist, Physical Therapy Orthopaedic Specialists, Inc., Minneapolis, Minnesota; Clinical Assistant Professor, Program in Physical Therapy, University of Tennessee, Memphis, Tennessee

Marla M. Bookhout, M.S., P.T.
Physical Therapist, and Clinical Coordinator, Postgraduate Internship Program, Physical Therapy Orthopaedic Specialists, Inc., Minneapolis, Minnesota

Edwin Dale, Ph.D.
Associate Professor, Department of Gynecology-Obstetrics, Emory University School of Medicine, Atlanta, Georgia

Hollis Herman, M.S., R.P.T.
Lecturer, Department of Physical Therapy, Northeastern University, Boston, Massachusetts

Joseph Kahn, Ph.D., P.T.
Clinical Assistant Professor of Electrotherapy, State University of New York at Stony Brook Health Sciences Center, Physical Therapy Program, Stony Brook, New York; Adjunct Associate Professor, Physical Therapy Division, Touro College, Huntington, New York; Clinical Associate, Physical Therapy Program, New York University, New York, New York.

Rhonda K. Kotarinos, M.S., P.T.
President, Women's Therapeutic Services, Ltd., Melrose Park, Illinois

Valerie C. Lee, M.A.
Research Coordinator, Melpomene Institute for Women's Health Research, Minneapolis, Minnesota

Michael K. Lindsay, M.D.
Assistant Professor, Department of Gynecology-Obstetrics, Emory University School of Medicine, Atlanta, Georgia

Judy Mahle Lutter, M.A.
President, Melpomene Institute for Women's Health Research, Minneapolis, Minnesota

Karen M. Mullinax, C.N.M., M.N.
Assistant Professor, Nurse Midwifery Program, Department of Community Health, Emory University School of Medicine; Staff Nurse Midwife, Grady Hospital, Atlanta, Georgia

C. Anne Patterson, M.D.
Assistant Professor, Department of Gynecology-Obstetrics; Collaborative Scientist, Yerkes Regional Primate Research Center, Emory University School of Medicine, Atlanta, Georgia

Pamela Shrock, R.P.T., Ph.D., A.C.C.E.
National Faculty Member, American Society for Psycho-prophylaxis in Obstetrics (ASPO), Arlington, Virginia; Perinatal Health Educator, McGaw Medical Center of Northwestern University; Psychotherapist and Staff Therapist, Adult Sexuality Program, McGaw Medical Center of Northwestern University, Chicago, Illinois

Yvette Woodrow, B.P.T.
Lecturer, School of Physical Therapy, University of Saskatchewan College of Medicine, Saskatoon, Saskatchewan, Canada; Formerly, National Chairman, Division of Obstetrics, Canadian Physiotherapy Association, Ontario, Canada

Preface

> Physical therapists practicing in obstetrics are certainly specialists. Some
> of them are nationally eminent. Mostly they received their certification
> and function under the auspices of other organizations. As a result, many
> have seen their vocation as an alternative to P.T. rather than an integral
> part of it.*

With the above statement in mind, the primary purpose of this book is to
provide the educator, student, and practicing physical therapist with a single
foundational and comprehensive professional source on current obstetric and
gynecologic physical therapy practice. While a majority of the contributing
authors are physical therapists with experience in clinical practice, research,
administration, and education, others are physicians, exercise physiologists,
nurse midwives, and researchers in the field of women's health issues. My
approach to clinical problem solving is to consider the continuum of normal to
abnormal (or function to dysfunction). The flow of the book follows this format
to provide the reader with the tools needed for study, practice, and education.
Educators, students, and practicing therapists at different points in their
respective endeavors will be able to access needed information relative to
major issues in obstetric and gynecologic practice. To encourage additional
research of specific topic areas, numerous references are included.

In Chapter 1, the normal physiologic adjustments to pregnancy are
examined; the chapter serves as a foundation for critical analysis of clinical and
research issues presented later in the book. For example, in Chapter 7, the
controversy regarding the use of exercise in pregnancy, in both human and
animal studies, is discussed by an exercise physiologist and a nurse midwife.
The authors of Chapter 8 present exercise data of pregnant women with a
history of significant and consistent prepregnancy activity levels, including
athletic training. Both chapters provide insight into clinical decision making
and guidelines one might use when giving an exercise prescription.

---

* Noble E: Petition to the Board of Directors, American Physical Therapy Association, for the
proposed Section on Obstetrics and Gynecology, March 1977.

Chapters 2, 3, and 4 provide a format for the evaluation and management of muscoloskeletal problems during pregnancy. In Chapter 2 lumbopelvic and upper quarter dysfunction are considered; although entire books have been written on this topic, unique to this chapter is its concentration on the modifications necessary to treat the pregnant client. Chapters 3 and 4 cover diastasis recti and urogenital dysfunctions, whose management is critical to a comprehensive approach to the pregnant client. Chapter 3 includes original research findings from both authors' recent graduate experiences in diastasis recti delineation and management, and Chapter 4 gives special emphasis to pelvic floor dysfunction and management.

In Chapter 5 the reader is provided with a review of electrical modalities employed in the treatment of obstetric and gynecologic clients. The controversy surrounding the use of electrical modalities for specific conditions such as during labor is briefly considered.

In Chapters 6 and 9, the physical therapist's role in the development and provision of childbirth education programs is discussed. While Chapter 6 examines the use of specific relaxation techniques and their integration into the overall educational format, Chapter 9 explores the issues of providing quality childbirth education to "adult learners" with varied backgrounds and needs.

While working on this editorial project, I was supported, in part, by a Maternal and Child Health Training grant, awarded by the U.S. Department of Health and Human Services, Bureau of Health Care Delivery and Assistance. I am grateful to Pamela Catlin, Richard Nyberg, and Linda Woodruff for their editorial assistance, and especially to Denise Smith, my right hand, whose typing, editing, and organizational assistance made my job easier. I appreciate Suzanne Campbell for prodding me to take on this project, and I am indebted to Jim Little for providing me with a good role model during my early childbirth education training. I am personally thankful to Robert Bradley, who taught me and constantly reminds me about the natural wonder of birth, to Elizabeth Noble for her vision, expertise, and goal-related persistence, and lastly to Al Hallum, who so caringly supported my family in our overwhelming birthing experience.

Elaine Wilder, R.P.T., M.A.C.T.

Contents

1 | Maternal Physiology in Pregnancy

C. Anne Patterson
Michael K. Lindsay

Every cell, tissue, organ, and system of the maternal organism is influenced by pregnancy. Certain of these influences are too subtle and presumably insignificant to be detected by contemporary technology. Others are much more dramatic, easily detected, and play a significant role in the physiologic economy of the maternal-fetal complex. It is the intent of this chapter to provide an overview of the anatomic and physiologic changes which occur in the maternal system during the childbearing year and to further relate these changes to an imposed exercise or health program which may be existing concurrently. This approach is intended to be informative and at the same time to address many contemporary questions that are being raised concerning the effects of exercise during pregnancy. The overall goal of this chapter and Chapter 2 is to demonstrate that pregnancy, while admittedly a radical departure from the physiologic and anatomic normal, is regulated by the hormonic mechanisms of the body and is usually a normal variant. Pregnancy is not a contraindication to maintenance of personal fitness unless exacerbated by physical or medical disease. When coupled with a healthful lifestyle, including exercise and nutrition, pregnancy can result in both a healthy mother and a healthy infant.

The anatomic and physiologic maternal alterations during the childbearing year that are described below represent only the major and presumably significant changes which occur in all healthy pregnancies. The descriptions are not intended to be exhaustive, and the reader is referred to standard textbooks of obstetrics for additional details. The focus of this presentation is naturally a reflection of our interests and biases. Additionally, we feel that the changes described herein are the most important relative to the impact of exercise on pregnancy, as will be discussed in Chapter 7. Finally, we have taken the prerogative of describing certain clinical changes that occur during pregnancy, and have attempted to relate them in a meaningful manner to the underlying anatomic and physiologic changes.

The sum of the anatomic, physiologic, and biochemical changes which occur during the 280-day span of human pregnancy are, in a word, profound. One of the most subtle yet extremely critical biochemical changes involves the production of human chorionic gonadatropin (hCG) by the trophoblast, which then stimulates the pre-existing corpus luteum to continue its production of estrogen and progesterone. This is essential in order to maintain the uterine endometrium as a site favorable for continued implantation, nourishment, and development of the recently fertilized egg. The unseen hormone changes are no less important or dramatic than the thousandfold increase in size which occurs in the maternal uterus at term, bulging with its multi-billion cell 3500 g infant that has arisen from the fusion of two single celled gametes some 10 lunar months earlier. These profound physiologic adaptations to pregnancy represent exquisite biochemical interactions that focus to insure the production of the newest member of the species. Equally astounding is the fact that in approximately ninety days after delivery that same maternal system returns to its pre-pregnancy anatomic and physiologic state, again with many obvious as well as subtle adaptations.

The most obvious adaptations (reproductively speaking) are those changes which occur in the female reproductive system in response to the presence of a normal intra-uterine pregnancy. To the observer, changes in body conformation, skin texture, mood, temperament, and personality may be the most obvious changes. To the physiologist, the adaptations of the cardio-respiratory system are the most important, and the hematologist notes the dramatic changes in blood volume, iron requirements, and alterations in hematocrit and coagulation. The endocrinologist is impressed with alterations in thyroid function, ovarian and placental hormones, and the endocrine mechanisms of the induction of labor, whereas the physical therapist attaches importance to musculoskeletal changes, diastasis recti abdominas, and other adaptations. Each topic addressed will help the physical therapist gain a more complete understanding of the physiologic changes that occur during gestation. Some topics may be omitted, as information is lacking or the changes are not significant. If a favorite system has been ignored, it is due to an oversight by the author and does not reflect the importance of that system. All changes are discussed as they relate to their importance during pregnancy or to the effects of the impact of exercise on that pregnancy.

THE ENDOCRINE SYSTEM

Human Chorionic Gonadotropin

Immediately upon implantation of the fertilized egg into the estrogen-progesterone stimulated uterine endometrium, the ovaries cease their function of producing a monthly membrane follicle. At the same time, the corpus luteum

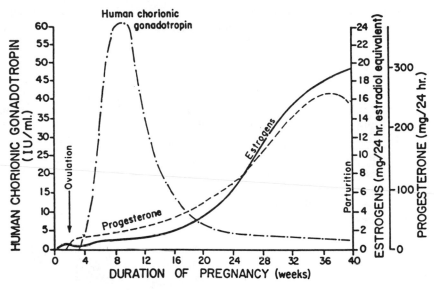

Fig. 1-1. Rates of secretion of estrogens, progesterone, and chorionic gonadotropin at different stages of pregnancy. (Guyton AC: Textbook of Medical Physiology. 6th Ed. WB Saunders, Philadelphia, 1981.)

of the ovum that was fertilized begins to be stimulated by hCG, which is produced and secreted by the developing extra-embryonic trophoblast. This hCG production can be detected in the serum within 10 days of conception. The production rises rapidly and peaks between the eighth and tenth week of pregnancy, then falls to a level that is maintained for the duration of the pregnancy (Fig. 1-1). The peak persists for longer periods of time in multiple gestations and in abnormal conditions. After delivery, detectable hCG disappears from the serum in 7 to 10 days.

High hCG levels function to maintain a favorable environment for implantation and development of the early embryo. This is accomplished by inducing the production of estrogen and progesterone by the corpus luteum. The level of these hormones is critical for the maintenance of the pregnancy until the placenta is mature enough to produce the required steroid hormones. After this time the amount of hCG in the serum falls to its steady state level.

Human Placental Lactogen

Another hormone elaborated by trophoblastic tissue which is unique during pregnancy is human placental lactogen, (hPL). It is also known as human chorionic somatomamotropin. Its elaboration begins about the fifth week of pregnancy and increases progressively throughout the remainder of gestation. This hormone has several effects on the fetus and it has important effects on the glucose and fat metabolism of the mother. It causes a decrease in utilization of glucose by the mother and an increase in the glucose available to the fetus. The hormone also promotes release of free fatty acids in the mother.

Estrogen

The placenta, like the corpus luteum, secretes both estrogen and progesterone. The amount of estrogen produced during pregnancy is seen in Figure 1-1. By the end of gestation the increase in production is about 30 times normal.

Estrogen exerts its effect mainly on reproductive and associated organs. This increased quantity of estrogen causes enlargement of the uterus, breast, and external genitalia. It also exerts a relaxing effect on various pelvic ligaments. This causes the sacroiliac joints to become relatively limber and the symphysis pubis to separate slightly and become more elastic.

Progesterone

Progesterone is also a hormone essential for pregnancy. It is secreted in small quantities by the corpus luteum at the onset of pregnancy. As the placenta matures progesterone is secreted in increasingly large quantities throughout pregnancy (Fig. 1-1). It has special effects that are essential for the normal progression of pregnancy.

Initially progesterone is essential for the nutrition of the early embryo. Progesterone also decreases the contractility of the gravid uterus and helps prepare the breasts for lactation.

THE REPRODUCTIVE SYSTEM

During pregnancy the component organs of the female reproductive tract undergo considerable change. These changes are not only important to the continuation of the pregnancy but also serve as clinical signs that obstetric health care providers can utilize in their management of the pregnancy.

Vagina and Vulva

Edema and increased vascularity affect the vagina and vulvar areas during pregnancy. The vagina as well as the perineal body become relaxed. This facilitates the delivery. As pregnancy advances, increased vascularity of the vulva is noted. The patient often feels as if she is "sitting on something." While this problem may be common, complications are rare. Both edema and increased vascularity regress totally after delivery.

Uterus

The uterus must adapt to contain the growing fetus and placenta. These changes include hypertrophy of the muscle coat, increased vascularity, development of the lower uterine segment, and softening of the cervix.

At term the uterus weighs about 1 kg and measures approximately 35 cm in length. In contrast, the nonpregnant uterus weighs around 60 grams. The pregnant uterus usually rotates on its long axis with the anterior surface usually facing slightly to the right. The fundus enlarges significantly during gestation; therefore, the entry of the fallopian tubes may lie well below the top of the uterus.

The growth of the myometrium is due to both distension and hormonal stimulation. In early pregnancy the enlargement is due to an increase in the number of cells, but in later pregnancy the enlargement is chiefly due to hypertrophy of the individual cells. By term each muscle cell is about ten times the length it was before pregnancy.

Cervix

The cervix also hypertrophies during pregnancy but not to the extent of the uterus. Increased vascularity is noted; this gives a bluish color to the cervix. The cervical canal is still present during gestation but it shortens. However, the internal os must remain intact to maintain the pregnancy.

Breast

Estrogen stimulation causes active growth and branching of the ductal tissue. It also causes thickening of the skin of the nipple. Progesterone effects the development of the glandular tissue. Similar changes occur during the menstrual cycle but to a much lesser degree. During pregnancy the net effect of the hormonal stimulation is that the breasts become more prominent. In fact, each breast may increase in weight by 500 mg.

The nipple becomes larger and more erectile. The areolar skin becomes more pigmented and slightly raised. If increased pigmentation occurs it will persist as a permanent change. Patchy streaks may occur on the outside of the areolar in dark skinned women. These secondary areolar disappear after delivery. Striae similar to those seen in the abdomen are often found in the skin over the breast.

Mammary tissue may be found at other sites in the body along the milk line. Most commonly this tissue is found in the axillae. Such breast tissue will enlarge during pregnancy and will frequently become tense and painful since there is inadequate drainage to the main duct system.

MUSCULOSKELETAL SYSTEM
Abdominal Wall

The muscles of the abdominal wall must stretch to accommodate the growing uterus. The stretching usually resolves after delivery in most women; however, in some multiparous women muscle tone is decreased. This often allows the uterus to sag forward. In some patients these changes are manifest by an umbilicus which may become flattened or even protrude. In other patients the abdominal wall muscles do not withstand the pressure of the uterus and the rectus muscles separate in the midline. This is known as diastasis recti. In severe cases the uterus is covered by only skin, fascia, and peritoneum. In rare instances herniation may occur through the diastasis when the patient stands.

The ligaments that help support the uterus must also stretch as the uterus grows. These changes may be associated with low abdominal pain or low back pain. However, patients do not always feel discomfort from these changes.

Pelvic Joints

Relaxation and some softening of the sacroiliac joints may occur during pregnancy. This may cause some pain in the hips or difficulty in walking. Similar changes may occur in the ligaments and fibrocartilage of the symphysis pubis leading to increased mobility of the joint. The mobility that occurs may lead to increased tenderness and in some patients, extraordinary soreness.

Posture

Postural changes occur throughout pregnancy due to the increase in size and weight of the gravid uterus. This type of change is called lumbar lordosis (Fig. 1-2). There is an increase in curvature of the lumbar spine because the enlarging uterus causes a shift in the patient's center of gravity. This causes the patient to lean backward to keep her balance and is frequently associated with the common complaint of low back pain.

THE INTEGUMENT

Skin changes vary considerably from patient to patient. An increase in pigmentation on the face in a mask-like distribution may occur. This is known as chloasma. This change usually disappears after delivery. Increased pigmentation of the areola of the breasts and the linea alba of the lower abdomen occur during pregnancy. Like the pigmentation of the areola the changes in the linea

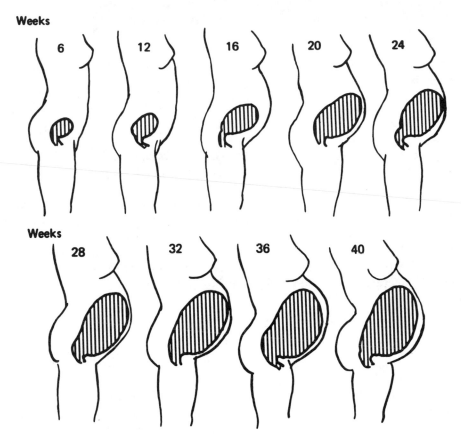

Fig. 1-2. Development of postural changes during pregnancy. (Quilligen EJ: Maternal physiology. p. 338. In Danforth DN (ed): Obstetrics and Gynecology. 4th Ed. Harper & Row, Philadelphia, 1982.)

alba can become permanent. This is why the linea alba may be referred to as the linea nigra.

In many patients a breakdown in the subcutaneous tissue over the abdomen occurs due to rupture of the elastic fibers in the skin. This change is commonly referred to as stretch marks or striae gravidarium. While stretching may be involved this is not the main problem. In fact, striae are not usually found in patients with abdominal distension from other causes, (e.g., ovarian tumors or ascites). They are seen in patients with Cushing's syndrome, a state where high glucocorticoid levels are found. A similar hormonal state is present during pregnancy and may affect the formation of striae.

The striae that form during pregnancy may appear pink, red, or purple. After delivery they become silvery-white. This change is often seen on the breast, inner thighs, and iliac crest as well.

CARDIOVASCULAR SYSTEM

The changes that develop in the cardiovascular system are quite remarkable because they occur over a short period of time and are completely reversible.

The Heart

The heart is pushed upward by the elevation of the diaphragm and rotated forward so that the apex beat is moved upward and laterally, appearing in the fourth rather than the fifth intercostal space.

The lateral displacement of the left border of the heart may give a somewhat exaggerated clinical impression of cardiac enlargement but the heart is indeed a little bigger in pregnancy. By radiologic measurement its volume increases by 70 to 80 ml (about 12 percent) between early and late pregnancy. It is still uncertain how much of the enlargement is due to the distention of the heart by increased diastolic filling and how much, if any, by muscle hypertrophy.

Cardiovascular Hemodynamics

Cardiac Output

Circumstantial evidence is strong that for the normal pregnant woman at rest (but not lying on her back), cardiac output rises within the first 10 weeks of pregnancy. It rises progressively (20–50 percent) above the nongravid level and an elevated cardiac output is maintained overall for the remainder of the pregnancy, although a slight decrease may occur near term. In twin pregnancy, mean cardiac output rises to a relatively stable plateau of 48 percent above the nongravid level.

During labor, cardiac output increases 20 to 30 percent with each uterine contraction in the first stage and as much as 50 percent with each contraction in the second stage. There is a marked increase in cardiac output immediately after delivery because of increased venous return to the heart following relief of uterine pressure on the inferior vena cava as well as contraction of the uterine vascular bed; this increment in cardiac output persists until the fourth postpartum day.

Heart Rate

The increased output of the heart is achieved by an increased heart rate and an increased stroke volume. Cardiac rate rises progressively throughout most of pregnancy with a plateau near term. A maximum increment of approximately 15 beats/min is noted near term, almost 20 percent above the nongravid level. In twin pregnancies the increase in cardiac rate is similar until

33 to 36 weeks gestation, when a marked surge to 40 percent above the nongravid level occurs. During labor, there is a marked and variable tachycardia.

Stroke Volume

Stroke volume increase is the single major factor responsible for increased cardiac output. Changes in stroke volume parallel changes in cardiac output, attaining a peak increment of 25 percent above the nongravid level in a singleton pregnancy and 38 percent above the nongravid level in a twin pregnancy. Postpartum, there is a marked increase in stroke volume which is maintained for 2 weeks.

Arterial Blood Pressure

Mean systolic blood pressure and mean diastolic blood pressure remain essentially unchanged during normal pregnancy except for a mild and transient decrease during the middle trimester. Both diastolic and systolic pressures decrease during the second trimester but rise to prepregnancy levels as term approaches.

Total Peripheral Resistance

The peripheral resistance of the circulation is calculated from the mean arterial blood pressure divided by the cardiac output. Since cardiac output is raised in pregnancy and arterial blood pressure is not, it follows that the resistance to flow—the peripheral resistance—must be decreased. The change is due to the establishment of new vascular beds and to a general relaxation of peripheral vascular tone.

Venous Pressure

Compared to those in arterial blood, changes in venous pressure during pregnancy can be relatively dramatic. The established pressure in the veins of the arm are not altered by pregnancy but pressures in the femoral and other leg veins are high. The femoral veins lead directly to the inferior vena cava and the heart without intervening valves so that with the subject horizontal, venous pressures from the legs to the heart are normally similar. In pregnancy there are three possible causes for venous obstruction:

1. Simple mechanical pressure by the weight of the uterus on both the iliac veins and the inferior vena cava.

2.   The pressure of the fetal head on the iliac veins.

3.   Hydrodynamic obstruction due to the outflow of blood at relatively high pressure from the uterus.

The high pressure in the femoral veins drops abruptly after delivery. Varicose veins of the legs and vulva and hemorrhoids may appear in pregnancy or are usually accentuated if present beforehand.

THE HEMATOLOGIC SYSTEM

The physiologic changes in the circulating blood during pregnancy and the puerperium are marked and show wide variation. There are dramatic changes in whole blood volume that affect hemoglobin, red cell indices, and the metabolism of iron. The hemostatic mechanisms show profound alterations compared with the nonpregnant state.

Plasma Value

It is now firmly established that plasma volume rises progressively throughout pregnancy to plateau in the last 8 weeks. Healthy women in a normal first pregnancy increase their plasma volume from a low-pregnant level of about 2600 ml by about 1250 ml. In subsequent pregnancies the increase is greater and may be about 1500 ml. Most of the increase takes place before 32–34 weeks gestation; thereafter there is relatively little change. The increase is related to the size of the fetus, and there are particularly large increases of plasma volume associated with multiple pregnancy.

Red Cell Mass

There is less published information on red cell mass than plasma volume and the results are more variable. The rise in red cell mass is about 18 percent for women not given iron medication in pregnancy and about 30 percent for those given iron. As with plasma volume the extent of the increase is likely to be related to the size of the conceptus. The red cell mass is reduced immediately at delivery as a result of blood loss and this is followed by a temporary erythroid hypoplasia until nonpregnant blood volumes are reached around 3 weeks after delivery. The hemoglobin, hematocrit, and red cell count decline during pregnancy because the expansion of plasma volume is greater than that of red cell mass.

Red Cell Production

There is evidence that red cell production is more rapid in pregnancy. The nature of the stimulus to red cell production is not known, but erythropoietin is thought to be involved. To maintain a higher level for hemoglobin, hematocrit, and red cell mass, supplemental iron must be given in a form that is readily absorbed. This may not be necessary in a well-nourished woman, but in the patient that has poor iron stores and inadequate nutrition, iron supplementation is essential.

The White Cells

The total white cell count rises in pregnancy. This is due to an increase of neutrophil polymorphonuclear leucocytes. The mean total white cell count is about 9,000 cells/mm^3 but can be as high as 15,000 cells per/mm^3. There is a further neutrophilia at the onset of labor even in uncomplicated pregnancies. The count returns to nonpregnant levels by 6 days postpartum. The metabolic activity of granulocytes is increased during pregnancy. The leucocyte alkaline phosphatase score rises from the nonpregnant state to reach levels in the third trimester which are usually encountered only during the course of significant infections while not pregnant. There is a fall in activity a few days before delivery and then a sharp rise during labor.

The lymphocyte count does not alter significantly during pregnancy and there is no change in the number of circulating T cells and B cells. However, factors in maternal serum suppress in vitro lymphocyte functions and cell-mediated immunity is profoundly depressed. There is no evidence of impairment of the production of immunoglobulin or of hormonal immunity. The depression of cell-mediated immunity during pregnancy may be relevant to the survival of the fetus.

RESPIRATORY SYSTEM

The purpose of breathing is to acquire oxygen, to deliver it to body tissues, and to eliminate carbon dioxide; the amounts depend on the demands of the body. Frequently measured respiratory functions (Fig. 1-3) are defined as follows:

1. Tidal volume: the volume of air inspired or expired in each respiration.
2. Inspiratory reserve volume: the maximum amount of air which can be inspired, beyond the normal tidal respiration.
3. Expiratory reserve volume: the maximum amount of air which can be expired after normal expiration.

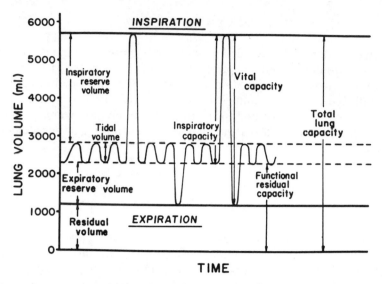

Fig. 1-3.   Respiratory excursions during normal breathing and during maximal inspiration and expiration. (Guyton AC: Textbook of Medical Physiology. 6th Ed. WB Saunders, Philadelphia, 1981.)

4. Residual volume: the volume of gas remaining in the lungs, not including the anatomic dead space of the tracheal and bronchial tree, at the end of maximal expiration.

5. Total lung capacity: the maximum volume to which the lungs can be expanded with the greatest possible inspiratory effort.

6. Inspiratory capacity: the tidal volume plus the inspiratory reserve volume. It is the maximum volume of air which can be inspired from the resting and expiratory position.

7. Functional residual capacity: the expiratory reserve volume plus the residual volume. It is the amount of air which remains in the lungs at the end of normal respiration.

8. Vital capacity: the maximum volume of gas which can be expired after a maximum inspiration. It is the inspiratory reserve volume plus the tidal volume plus the expiratory reserve volume.

During pregnancy the basal metabolic rate increases as well as the size of the patient. These changes increase the oxygen requirements of the mother. At term the amount of oxygen required is approximately 20 percent above normal. A corresponding increase in the expired amount of carbon dioxide is noted. Progesterone appears to act in concert, causing a central stimulation effect on the respiration center. This also effects the increase in respiratory effort and a subsequent reduction in PCO_2. These changes cause an increase in tidal

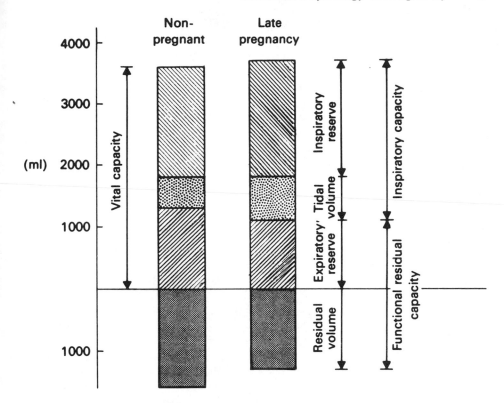

Fig. 1-4. Subdivisions of lung volume and their alterations in pregnancy. (de Swiet M: The respiratory system. In Hytten F, Chamberlain G (eds): Clinical Physiology in Obstetrics. Blackwell Scientific Publications, Oxford, 1980.)

volume and in minute ventilation (Fig. 1-4). Minute ventilation is the amount of air inspired in one minute or the tidal volume multiplied by the respiratory rate. This increase in minute ventilation is called the "hyperventilation of pregnancy.

Other changes are also noted. The functional residual capacity and the residual volume of air are decreased because of the elevation of the diaphragm. Airway conductance and lung compliance are relatively unaffected by pregnancy. The lung volume at which airways in the dependent parts of the lung begin to close during expiration is the closing volume. The change in the closing volume effected by pregnancy is uncertain. A mild respiratory alkalosis exists and this usually causes blood PCO_2 to be slightly lower than normal.

Dyspnea is common in pregnancy and can be experienced as early as 20 weeks gestation. The symptoms closely correlate with alveolar PCO_2 measurements, which reach their nadir in the late second trimester. In most patients who are evaluated because they complain of dyspnea a normal respiratory function is found for their given stage of gestation.

URINARY TRACT

Alterations in the urinary tract during pregnancy are quite profound. They may cause significant changes in the measured values of creatinine and blood urea nitrogen. Values considered normal in the nonpregnant woman may indicate impaired renal function in the pregnant state.

The earliest recognized morphologic changes in the urinary tract in pregnancy are the dilatations of the renal pelvis and ureters. The physiologic hydroureter of pregnancy is characterized by a marked increase in the diameter of the ureteral lumen. This is thought to be due to mechanical obstruction of the ureter by the uterus as the ureter crosses the pelvic brim. Hypotonicity and hypomotility of the musculature accompanies these changes. There is a right-sided preponderance of pyeloureteral dilatation above the pelvic brim which may be explained by the uterine dextrorotation. In addition to dilatation, the ureters elongate during pregnancy and become more tortuous. The ureters are also displaced laterally to some degree, especially in the second half of pregnancy, probably as a result of the growing uterus in the midline.

Several etiologies for the hydroureter of pregnancy have been considered. They include compression by the pregnant uterus, the iliac arteries, and the ovarian vein complexes. Research work in primates support a hormonal etiology for hydroureter. These experiments implicate the increased levels of progesterone, gonadotropins, and estrogens in pyeloureteral dilatation.

The smooth muscle relaxation caused by progesterone also affects the bladder. Estrogenic stimulation of the trigone causes hyperplasia and muscular hypertrophy. The bladder is displaced anteriorly and superiorly late in the second and during the third trimesters. The bladder mucosa becomes congested and the size and tortiuosity of the blood vessels increase. There are no other major changes of the bladder mucosa during pregnancy.

The changes that occur normally during pregnancy may contribute to stasis of urine and in turn lead to urinary tract infection. In pregnancy there is an increased indicence of acute pyelonephritis and asymptomatic bacteriuria. The patient may complain of frequent micturition. This may be associated with infection or due to a decreased bladder capacity produced by the proximity of the developing fetus. Increased vascularity of the trigone of the bladder also contributes to the problem.

The urinary tract changes that occur during pregnancy resolve relatively rapidly postpartum. Most resolution occurs within the first 48 hours postpartum and by 3 months anatomic dimensions have returned to the pregestational values.

SUGGESTED READINGS

Bailey RR, Rolleston GL: Kidney length and ureteric dilatation in the puerperium. J Obstet Gynecol Br Commonw 55:78, 1971

Beydoun SN: Morphologic changes in the renal tract in pregnancy. Clin Obstet and Gynecol 28:249, 1986

Clayton SG, Lewis TLT, Pinker GI, Edward A: Obstetrics by Ten Teachers. 14th Ed. E Arnold, London, 1985

Creasy RK, Resnik R: Maternal Fetal Medicine. WB Saunders, Philadelphia, 1984

Danforth DN: Obstetrics and Gynecology. 4th Ed. Harper & Row, Philadelphia, 1982

Guyton AC: Textbook of Medical Physiology. 7th Ed. WB Saunders, Philadelphia, 1987

Hodson CJ: Radiographic kidney size. p. 136. In Black DAK (ed): Renal Disease. Blackwell Scientific Publications, Oxford, 1968

Prichard JA, MacDonald PC, Gehr NF: Williams Obstetrics. 17th Ed. Appleton-Century-Crofts, New York, 1984

de Swiet M: The Respiratory System. p. 79. In Hytten F, Chamberlain G (eds): Clinical Physiology in Obstetrics. CV Mosby, 1980

Van Nagenen G, Jenkins RH: An experimental examination of factors causing ureteral dilatation of pregnancy. J Urol 42:1010, 1939

2 | Physical Therapy Management of Musculoskeletal Disorders During Pregnancy

Marla M. Bookhout
William G. Boissonnault

Pregnancy is a time of increased vulnerability for the musculoskeletal system. Pre-existing dysfunctions are aggravated and new problems may be created by the changes that occur in a woman's body during the childbearing year. These changes include variation in center of gravity and posture, expansion of the rib cage with elevation of the diaphragm, weight gain, fluid retention, and softening of connective tissues due to hormonal changes. The pain and dysfunction which may accompany these changes can often be addressed by a physical therapist. This chapter gives an overview of the musculoskeletal problems encountered by the pregnant woman, followed by a review of the general principles of subjective and objective assessment and treatment. A detailed outline of specific upper quarter and lumbopelvic evaluation and treatment techniques is then presented, with particular emphasis on the modifications and precautions the physical therapist should be aware of for the pregnant patient.

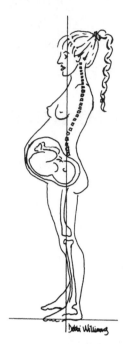

Fig. 2-1. As her uterus enlarges, the pregnant woman shifts her upper body weight over the pelvis to minimize displacement of her center of gravity.

OVERVIEW OF MUSCULOSKELETAL CHANGES DURING PREGNANCY

Postural Changes

As the uterus enlarges, the mother's center of gravity changes, usually affecting posture.[1-6] The increased weight low and anterior causes the woman to shift her upper body back over the pelvis to prevent falling forward (Fig. 2-1). Some authors report an increase in the forward head and shoulders posture,[2,6] while others describe elevation of the head and hyperextension of the cervical spine.[4] Most authors assume an increase in the lumbar lordosis accompanied by anterior rotation of the pelvis.[1,3,5,7] Fries and Hellebrandt, however, photographed the changing posture of a woman throughout her pregnancy and found "unexpectedly slight changes in the lumbar region." The major counterbalancing adjustments were made by elevating the head and extending the cervical spine while extending the knees and leaning back at the ankles.[4] If indeed a woman does increase her lumbar lordosis as her pregnancy progresses, pre-existing lumbar problems, which ordinarily are worsened by hyperextending the lumbar spine, may be aggravated.[6] Examples of such conditions are spondylolisthesis,[3] diffuse degenerative facet joint disease,[8] and lateral or subarticular recess stenosis.[9] Bushnell notes that an increase in the amount of lordosis at the thoracolumbar junction in pregnancy may cause

chanical stress on the muscles and ligaments in that area, causing foraminal
owing. He feels this may be responsible for radicular irritation manifesting
in along the course of the iliohypogastric and ilioinguinal nerves,
rly in the groin and pubic area as well as posteriorly from the
umbar junction to the ilia.[1]

pensatory thoracic kyphosis may occur as the lumbar lordosis in-
he enlarging breasts add to this postural strain, and radicular
an be experienced in the arms, chest, and head.[6] Maintenance of
ead and shoulders posture may lead to thoracic outlet syndrome
ise of the brachial plexus, the subclavian artery, and occasion-
an vein.[10]

Expansion of the Rib Cage

the transverse diameter of the chest increases and the
vated. The subcostal angle increases even before
erted on the ribs by the growing fetus.[2,11] The normal
become stretched over the first rib, which has
es "acroparasthesia," a variant of thoracic outlet
experiences pain, tingling, and numbness in the
chest circumference increases, pre-existing
ysfunctions may become mechanically aggra-

to Connective Tissue Changes

anges to which the musculoskeletal
the changes brought about by the
relaxin concentrations are highest
y playing a part in changing the
and facilitate delivery.[13] Serum
t trimester, remaining elevated
after delivery. No prelabor
man females.[13,14]

us laxity, soften cartilage,
es allow more stress to be
possibly causing strains
of the symphysis pu-
g pregnancy.[2,3,5,12,15-17]
rp and Fray in 1938
ts of 2 to 3 mm and
rage joint widt'
pubic wideni
d that primi

with measurable separation definitely had shorter labors than those without,
and that occiput posterior infants spontaneously turned more often in those
women with pubic separations of greater than 7 mm.[15]

In 1933 Boland reported 10 cases of pathologic separation of the symphysis
pubis during parturition, representing 1 in 685 deliveries. Four of these cases
followed normal delivery, but two were due to forceps delivery and two
occurred after women suffered falls during pregnancy. Boland noted that when
the pubis separated abnormally, the sacroiliac joint was involved on one or
both sides. He found that these women demonstrated low back pain, leg pain
and pain at the symphysis pubis, a waddling gait with positive Trendelenburg
sign, and weakness of hip motion.[16] Berezin described two types of "pelvic
insufficiency," which he defined as the inability of the pelvis to fulfill its
function as a supportive structure. He found that in some women the condition
occurred as a result of rupture of the pubic symphysis during delivery and in
others the symptomatic relaxation of the pelvic joints occurred during the last
half of pregnancy, apparently due to the increased relaxin levels. He noted that
most women recovered within 3 months after delivery, but symptoms increased prior to and during the menstrual period and were almost certain to
recur with subsequent pregnancies.[12] Other authors who have described
pathologic widening of the pubic symphysis also found involvement of
both sacroiliac joints, a condition cited as a cause for low back and lower
extremity pain.[3,5,15,17]

Weight Gain

The significant weight gain during pregnancy further increases the
strain on the already posturally and hormonally compromised
lumbar spine and pelvis, as well as the lower extremities. The
pronated feet may become more pronounced[6,7] and the hip and knee
ache with their increased load. Signs and symptoms of chondromalacia
are said to increase with pregnancy.[18] The combination of factors
probably causes a change in body mechanics during postural
activities such as stooping, bending and lifting increasing

Increased Fluid Retention

Besides weight gain, changes in the center of gravity, and increased ligamentous laxity, the pregnant woman must also deal with increased fluid retention, especially during the third trimester.[2] Various nerve compression syndromes are noted to occur during pregnancy due to the space-taking nature of edematous connective tissues.[18,23] Carpal tunnel syndrome occurs during pregnancy when swollen tissues compromise the median nerve as it passes through the tunnel formed by osseous and ligamentous structures on the volar side of the wrist. This causes pain, numbness, and tingling in the thumb and index and middle fingers.[23] Ulnar nerve compression may occur at the inner elbow or at Guyon's canal at the wrist, causing fourth and fifth finger symptoms. Thoracic outlet syndrome can occur due to swelling of the tissues in the scalene triangle, as well as in conjunction with the postural factors previously mentioned. As the feet and ankles become more swollen during pregnancy, posterior tibial nerve compression may occur in the tarsal tunnel posterior to the medial malleolus resulting in symptoms on the medial aspect of the foot.[18]

Although the musculoskeletal changes described here are expected during pregnancy, the problems that these changes may cause should not be ignored. The physical therapist is in an ideal position to evaluate musculoskeletal dysfunction and provide at least some measure of relief to the pregnant woman experiencing this condition.

PRINCIPLES OF ORTHOPEDIC EXAMINATION DURING PREGNANCY

The Position Paper for the Section on Obstetrics and Gynecology of the American Physical Therapy Association states that one of the functions of the physical therapist as a clinical practitioner in obstetrics/gynecology (ob/gyn) is to conduct a musculoskeletal evaluation of the obstetric patient.[24] The principles of musculoskeletal examination for the obstetric patient are the same as for any other patient. What makes the obstetric population clinically unique are the structural and physiologic changes that occur during the childbearing year. These changes have an effect on the choice of examination and treatment techniques, as well as on expected findings. For example, certain patient positions commonly used for evaluation should be avoided during various stages of pregnancy. From approximately the third month through delivery the patient should not be positioned prone since the growing fetus is no longer protected by the bony pelvis.[25] This position may also have to be avoided postpartum as well if the woman has undergone a caesarean section or has breast tenderness. During the third trimester, as the uterus shifts posteriorly and comes to rest on the vertebral column, the supine position should also be used with caution, since it could possibly cause partial occlusion of the inferior vena cava. This occlusion has a potentially harmful effect on the mother and the fetus.[26,27] Elevation of the patient's right side to an angle of approximately 30 degrees or greater in the supine position appears to sufficiently relieve the compression forces to allow normal blood flow, thus making possible the clinical use of this position. If the fetus is of sufficient size, it may be necessary to consider this positional precaution during the second trimester.

The general objectives of any orthopedic examination include finding the source or sources of the patient's symptoms, determining the stage of healing of the lesion (acute, subacute, or chronic condition), and discovering any associated dysfunction which may be directly or indirectly influencing the patient's problem. Developing a comprehensive treatment program for each patient is dependent on obtaining this information via the subjective and objective portions of the examination.

Subjective Examination

Minimal additions to the standard subjective examination scheme are necessary when evaluating the obstetric patient. Questions should be asked relating to illnesses or diseases common during pregnancy, and pre- and postnatal complications should be noted. General subjective examination principles as well as issues specific to the obstetric population will be addressed in this section.

Carrying out a complete and concise patient interview is important for the organization of the objective examination, overall assessment of the patient, and development of the proper treatment program. While each clinician will develop his or her own method and style for conducting the subjective examination, all clinicians should attempt to obtain certain specific information. This includes a precise description of the patient's chief complaints, noting the symptoms and the exact location. The behavior of each symptom should next be investigated by documenting whether the symptom is of constant or intermittent nature in general, as well as over a 24-hour period. This information may help determine whether the problem is mechanical (musculoskeletal) or nonmechanical in origin, a major consideration for the therapist. Generally, symptoms from a mechanical problem can be altered by certain movements or body/limb positions. Symptoms from visceral dysfunction or serious pathology may not be affected by movement position. As a general rule, pelvic disease may result in referred pain to the sacral region, while lower abdominal diseases may cause referred pain to the lumbar region. Back pain may be the only overt patient complaint in the presence of these diseases.[28,29] Relating movements or activity level to aggravation of the symptom, plus monitoring the time it takes for the symptom intensity to return to its original level, falls within the concept of irritability.[30] All of the above ideas related to symptom behavior should be applied to each of the patient's described symptoms.

Once current symptom behavior has been determined, a chronological history of the patient's problem should be explored, including original onset of symptoms, mechanism of injury (if trauma has occurred), previous history of similar episodes, and previous treatment and its resultant outcome. The remainder of the subjective examination should consist of a series of questions related to age, general health, and past medical history, including previous illnesses, injuries, or surgeries. Questions regarding past pregnancies and deliveries, medication currently being taken, and a general description of the patient's occupation are also important. As mentioned earlier, determining the mechanical versus nonmechanical origin of the patient's symptoms is extremely important. Some visceral disease processes may refer pain to the lumbosacral area. For example, acute pyelonephritis is one of the most common medical complications of pregnancy, with pain in the lumbar region being a common associated complaint. General questions should be included regarding associated symptoms, such as fever, urinary frequency and urgency, nausea, and vomiting.[25] Questions regarding past pregnancies and deliveries are important since complications from previous pregnancies may be related to the patient's current problem. Investigating complications of the current pregnancy or recent delivery may reveal important information about the musculoskeletal system which may impact on the objective examination or treatment. Prenatally, the patient should be questioned about such conditions as premature uterine contractions, incompetent cervix, or episodic uterine bleeding. The presence of any of these conditions may restrict or limit the woman's activities, including certain exercises. If urinary stress incontinence is present, the pelvic floor should be examined, as laxity may be a contributing factor.[31] Postnatally, questions should be asked regarding labor or delivery interventions, such as regional anesthetic injection, forceps delivery, episiotomy, or caesarean section. Specific musculoskeletal tissues may be compromised during these procedures and require treatment. Knowing what medication the patient is currently taking is helpful since side effects from the drugs may explain some of the patient's symptoms. In addition, since the prescribing of many medications is halted or dosages dramatically reduced during pregnancy, the clinician needs to know which medications were taken prior to the pregnancy and for what reasons.

The information obtained during the subjective examination must be correlated with the objective examination findings before assessment of the patient's problem can be completed. The patient interview can be difficult and time consuming if it is not conducted in an organized fashion. To help keep the interview progressing in an organized and controlled fashion, the therapist should tell the patient that a series of questions will be asked in a specific order, after which the patient will have the opportunity to discuss any important information not already addressed.

Objective Examination

Objective examination findings help the therapist determine the source or sources of the patient's symptoms, the stage of wound healing, and areas of dysfunction which need to be treated. Identifying the location of the lesion based solely on the symptomatic area described by the patient can be misleading, as pain and neurologic signs are often present at a distance from the site of irritation. Therefore, the clinician should perform tests designed to alter the patient's symptoms. Provoking tenderness or soreness is not enough; the *specific* pain or the tingling etc. must be altered in order to locate the lesion accurately. By performing the tests carefully and precisely and by correlating the positive signs (tests which alter symptoms) with the negative signs (tests which do not alter symptoms), one may be able to localize the lesion to a specific structure or area. This information allows the therapist to direct treatment to the appropriate region. Deciding if the lesion is in the acute, subacute, or chronic stage of wound healing is important since this information dictates how conservative or aggressive the treatment should be. Symptom irritability and the presence or absence of the cardinal signs of inflammation are pieces of information which help the clinician determine the stage of wound healing. The most important piece of the puzzle is dysfunction. The assessed dysfunction directly and/or indirectly related to the lesion dictates precisely which treatment should be utilized. Examples of dysfunction may include joint hypo- or hypermobility and soft tissue imbalances, including weak muscles and/or shortened, tight structures, all of which may result in abnormalities found during the static postural and dynamic movement components of the examination.

Objective assessment of dysfunction includes observing static and dynamic postures, palpating position and condition of tissues, testing both active and passive mobility, assessing length and mobility of soft tissues, and using resistance for provocation and to test muscle strength.

Observation of Static Posture and Gait

Observation of static posture and gait are initial components of the examination. Even though the postural changes previously described are expected in the pregnant woman, one may have to incorporate treatment to control these changes in order to help relieve a woman's symptoms. In addition to observation of posture and gait, the therapist should also note other changes important to the assessment of the patient, such as muscle atrophy, edema, and the redness associated with inflammation.

Bony and Soft Tissue Palpation

Bony and soft tissue palpation follows observation. As well as provoking painful structures, palpation allows the clinician to detect abnormal bone position and soft tissue texture which gives important information regarding areas of dysfunction.[32,33] During the last trimester the soft tissues of the trunk may become so stretched due to the increased size of the fetus that a considerable increase in soft tissue tension/tautness may be noted. The degree of tension could be considered abnormal in other patient populations. In addition, edema of the soft tissues, a common palpatory finding during pregnancy, is often associated with peripheral nerve entrapment problems.[23]

Active Motion Testing

Active range of motion should be assessed next. Based on active movement findings, the clinician can decide if passive or resisted testing should be attempted and if so, with what degree of caution. When assessing active range of motion, quantity and quality of movement should be considered, as well as provocation. When assessing the amount of movement in a pregnant woman, one needs to consider that the hormonal changes associated with pregnancy may result in more movement than usual. If active motion is restricted, passive testing will help the clinician determine what the restricting elements are. Dysfunction is suggested when a patient demonstrates abnormal quality of movement even though normal quantity of motion may be present. For example, a patient might forward bend fully, but midway through the movement the trunk might sharply deviate to the left and then return to the midline to complete the movement. Even though the patient has a normal amount of motion, forward bending is abnormal—a positive clinical sign. As with other tests, active movements may provoke the patient's symptoms. If so, when correlated with the other active, passive, and resisted test findings, it may be possible to determine which structure or region is involved.[29] This information would allow treatment of the appropriate area.

Passive Motion Testing

Documentation of quantity, quality, and provocation are important with passive testing also. For recording amount of passive range of motion with segmental testing of the spine and accessory movements of the extremities, the zero to six scale can be used.[34] During pregnancy, increased range of passive motion with both physiologic and accessory movement testing may be present due to hormonal changes. Quality of passive movement includes "endfeel," defined by Cyriax as the different sensations imparted to the tester's hands at the end of the possible range.[29] The different sensations may indicate which type of tissue is limiting the particular motion. This information helps the clinician decide which treatment technique to employ. A spasm endfeel or pain provoked before resistance is encountered suggests an acute condition. Pain provoked after the initial point of resistance during the passive movement suggests that the wound is in the chronic stage of healing and more aggressive treatment can be initiated.[29]

Resistance Testing

Information from resistance testing can be placed under three general categories: myotome testing for assessing neurologic status; muscle performance, including manual muscle testing; and provocation of the patient's symptoms. Assessing neurologic status is important for any patient population but especially so for the obstetric patient due to the common occurrence of thoracic outlet syndrome and peripheral nerve entrapment problems. Correlation of the myotome and manual muscle test results may help the clinician decide if the nerve lesion is central or peripheral in origin. Considering all of the postural changes and abnormalities which may be found in the obstetric population, manual muscle testing is an important part of one's examination.

Correlating the muscle groups which are weak with those which are tight or overstretched is important for the development of a comprehensive treatment program. These soft tissue imbalances are examples of dysfunction which can have a direct affect on the patient's condition. In the extremities, utilizing an isometric contraction of specific muscle groups around the joint allows one to primarily stress the myofascial unit. The clinician documents relative strength and provocation during these tests, which may help determine the specific muscle or muscles, involved and to what degree they have been damaged.[29]

Sensory and reflex testing, which are components of the neurologic examination, should also be included in the objective examination. These tests, along with the myotome and manual muscle testing results, will help the clinician determine which nerves, peripheral or central, are involved. Numerous special tests for each region of the body could be included in an examination, but it is not within the scope of this chapter to include them all. Some of these tests will be discussed as they relate to the clinical problems covered in the following sections of the chapter.

GENERAL PRINCIPLES OF TREATMENT FOR MUSCULOSKELETAL DYSFUNCTION DURING PREGNANCY

As with other patient populations, specific examination findings will dictate the makeup of the treatment program for the obstetric patient. All aspects of patient management for orthopedic problems apply to women during the childbearing year. Musculoskeletal dysfunction can become symptomatic any time during pregnancy, but generally the earlier in her pregnancy a woman is treated, the better the chance of successful management of her condition. As the pregnancy proceeds into the third trimester, extensive anatomic and physiologic changes may decrease the chances of therapeutic changes being made or maintained during treatment.

For relief of symptoms stemming from mechanical disorders of the musculoskeletal system, the dysfunction must ultimately be treated. There are times, though, when pain and associated muscle spasm or guarding may prevent direct treatment of the dysfunction. Numerous manual techniques and modalities are available to the clinician for pain management and muscle relaxation.

Joint dysfunction is a common clinical finding during pregnancy. Direct treatment of dysfunction may include improving joint mobility by various manipulation techniques[35] or stabilizing the joint with strengthening exercises and/or an external support. In the presence of hypermobility, treating any adjacent spinal segmental hypomobility[32] and/or soft tissue imbalance is important to decrease the mechanical stress on the involved segments during movements and static postures.

Dysfunction of soft tissue structures such as muscles, fascia, and skin can result in or accentuate static postural abnormalities and/or improper movement patterns. Poor movement patterns and postural alignment place added stress on the joints of the lumbar spine and pelvis, which are already abnormally stressed due to the postural and hormonal changes and weight gain associated with pregnancy. Soft tissue imbalances, with associated muscle weakness and/or tightness, are common clinical findings during pregnancy. For instance, weakness of the abdominals (upper and lower), hip extensors, and hip abductors is often present, accompanied by decreased flexibility of hip and trunk musculature, such as hip flexors, adductors, and hamstrings. These muscles are essential for normal patterns of movement and for good trunk and pelvic alignment during static postures such as standing.[36] Treatment of these imbalances includes appropriate strengthening and stretching exercises. According to Janda, attempting to strengthen weak muscles without stretching tight muscle groups in the area could result in an enhancement of the imbalance. In addition, he suggests that stretching exercises be initiated prior to strengthening exercises, based on the observation that weakened muscles occasionally spontaneously regain strength after tight antagonistic groups have been stretched.[37] Ideally, if women participate in prenatal exercise programs, the development of soft tissue imbalances may be prevented or already existing imbalances reduced, thereby decreasing the stresses on the lumbar spine and pelvic joints. (Such exercise programs should be designed to meet the individual needs of each participant.) Dysfunction of soft tissue structures can also be treated with various massage and myofascial release techniques. Movement therapy, such as the Feldenkrais, Alexander, and Aston Patterning approaches, augment stretching and strengthening exercises for the purpose of enhancing movement patterns and postural support.

Making the patient responsible for her own health is a key to successful management. If the patient is not following a comprehensive home exercise program or taking safety precautions, such as using proper body mechanics at home and work, maintaining any of the positive results achieved during the clinical visits will be difficult.

Numerous evaluation and treatment techniques are described by physical therapists and osteopaths for management of musculoskeletal dysfunction.[29,30,33,35,37-49] In the following section, techniques will be discussed that have been found to be most useful in the clinic. The biggest challenge facing the clinician is assessing and treating dysfunction without compromising the mother or fetus. Due to the fact that lower quarter dysfunction is much more common during pregnancy, less emphasis will be placed on the upper quarter.

UPPER QUARTER EXAMINATION AND MANAGEMENT FOR THE OBSTETRIC PATIENT

Very few technique modifications need to be made when doing an upper quarter examination of a pregnant woman. Most of the tests can be carried out in the sitting position, which does not compromise the fetus. If sitting is contraindicated, based on the patient's history, then positional modifications must be considered, as described earlier.

The following is a list describing a suggested upper quarter examination scheme, outlined by position.

I. Standing
  A. Observation
    1. Head position on neck
    2. Head/neck position on thorax
    3. Shoulder girdle position on thorax
    4. Upper extremity position
    5. Thorax position on pelvis
    6. Pelvis position on lower extremities
    7. Lower extremity position
    8. Foot positions plus arch status
    9. Note the presence of muscle atrophy, hypertrophy, edema, scar
  B. Palpation
    1. Soft tissue
      a. Temporalis, masseter muscles
      b. Cervical spine muscles (anterior, posterior, lateral)
      c. Scapular muscles
      d. Anterior shoulder girdle muscles (including pectoralis major and minor)
      e. Lymph nodes (submandibular, superficial parotid, occipital, superficial cervical)[50]
      f. Pulses (brachial, radial)
      g. Muscle tone, temperature, skin moisture, edema
    2. Bony
      a. Mastoid processes, nuchal line
      b. Hyoid bone
      c. Clavicle levels
      d. First rib position
      e. Acromium levels
      f. Scapula positions

      g. Spinous processes (cervical and thoracic spines)

      h. Bony landmarks

II. Sitting

   A. Active range of motion

     1. Mandibular depression; observe and palpate temporomandibular joints

     2. C1–2 rotation

     3. Cervical spine (forward/backward bending, side bending, rotation)

     4. Cervical distraction/compression (Fig. 2-2)

     5. Shoulder girdle elevation/depression

     6. Shoulder abduction, external and internal rotation

     7. Elbow, wrist, finger flexion and extension

   B. Neurologic examination (repeat in supine if positive)

     1. Sensation (dermatome)

     2. Motor (myotome)

     3. Reflexes

   C. Passive range of motion

     1. Cervical spine

     2. Cervicothoracic junction

     3. Thoracic spine, including ribs

   D. Special tests

     1. Brachial plexus stretch

     2. Foraminal closure

     3. Adson's maneuver

     4. Costoclavicular position

     5. Hyperabduction

III. Supine/Prone

   A. Palpation; repeat muscle and bony palpation as applicable

   B. Passive range of motion

     1. Cervical spine

     2. Cervicothoracic junction

     3. Thoracic spine, including ribs

     4. Shoulder girdle (scapulothoracic, acromioclavicular, sternoclavicular joints)

     5. Glenohumeral joint

     6. Muscle length (pectoralis major and minor, latissimus dorsi)

     7. Soft tissue mobility

Examination Techniques

General observation, including a postural examination, is the initial component of the evaluation. Abnormalities may clue the therapist in on the regions of the upper quarter which should be inspected more closely. Soft tissue palpation should include the lymph nodes, which, if palpable or

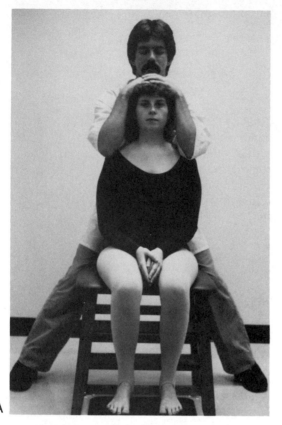

Fig. 2-2. (A) Cervical compression as a provocation test for the weight bearing structures of the neck. (*Figure continues.*)

A

thickened, may suggest the presence of infection. Bony palpation may indicate abnormal position (one sign of dysfunction), but position alone may be misleading in the presence of bony anomalies. Bony levels of the pelvis and femur should be assessed and lower quarter postural inspection performed to rule out potential lower quarter influence on the upper quarter structures.

Active range of motion assessment should include mandibular depression. One should observe and palpate the movement to detect joint dysfunction. If the movement is positive for dysfunction, a more detailed craniofacial examination can be carried out. Cervical spine rotation can be isolated to the atlantoaxial segment if tested with the head and neck bent forward. Rotation of the cervical spine with the neck in a neutral position can provide the initial vertebral artery test and allow an assessment of range of motion. If the active movements are negative, then overpressure can be added to further stress the area.

Many positions can be used for assessing passive range of motion. Passive movements can be of two types, physiologic and accessory. Examples of physiologic movements (movements which can be reproduced voluntarily)

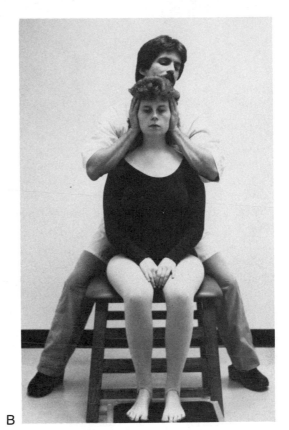

Fig. 2-2. (*Continued*). **(B)** Cervical distraction unweights the weight bearing structures of the neck.

B

include forward bending, rotation, etc. Examples of accessory movements (those which cannot be reproduced voluntarily) include central and unilateral pressures on a vertebrae, as described by Maitland.[30]

Cervical compression is a maneuver which primarily stresses the weight bearing structures of the neck (Fig. 2-2A). These structures include vertebral bodies, discs, uncovertebral joints, and facet joints. Cervical distraction (Fig. 2-2B) unweights the weight bearing structures and if the maneuver relieves the patient's symptoms, traction may be indicated for treatment. Selected active movements of the shoulder girdle, shoulder, elbow, wrist, and hand can be assessed. If any of the movements are positive, a more detailed examination of the area can be carried out. If portions of the neurologic examination are positive in the sitting weight bearing position, the test should be repeated in the supine nonweight bearing position. (The clinician should remember to place a pillow under the right buttocks of the pregnant woman). If the results change with position of the patient, specific positions for treatment may be indicated. Special tests will be addressed in the following section on thoracic outlet syndrome (TOS).

Thoracic Outlet Syndrome

Thoracic outlet syndrome is a common upper quarter problem found in the obstetric patient population. The onset of TOS or the aggravation of a pre-existing problem during pregnancy may be related to the upper quarter postural changes associated with pregnancy. Specifically, the development of increased forward head posture (FHP) may lead to compromise of the neurovascular structures associated with TOS. The forward head posture has many potential positional components, including backward bending of the upper cervical spine, increased kyphosis of the lower cervical and upper thoracic spine, elevation of the first rib, and internal rotation of the glenohumeral joints.[10] During pregnancy, the increased weight of the breasts,[51] compensation for an increased lumbar lordosis,[6] and abnormal costal patterns for respiration[7] may contribute to these upper quarter postural changes.

The term thoracic outlet syndrome implies compromise of the brachial plexus, subclavian artery, and possibly the subclavian vein, with associated symptoms radiating to the upper extremity. The most common sites of entrapment are the triangle consisting of the anterior and middle scalenes and the first rib, the area between the clavicle and first rib, and the area deep in the pectoralis minor where it attaches to the coracoid process. Grant's *Atlas of Anatomy*[52] and CIBA's pamphlet, *Thoracic Outlet Syndrome*,[53] are good pictorial references for these regions. Rhodes states that during pregnancy, TOS is primarily caused by the stretching of the neurovascular bundle over the elevated first rib.[7] The first rib may be elevated by the increased muscle activity of the anterior and middle scaleni. Hyperactivity of the scaleni may be caused by cervical spine dysfunction, excessive FHP, and upper respiratory patterns of breathing. First rib elevation may compromise the brachial plexus and subclavian vessels by increasing the tensile stress on the structures or by decreasing the available space for the structures between the first rib and clavicle. The underlying cause of the hyperactive scaleni must be treated if the elevated first rib problem is to be corrected. The abnormal muscle activity of the anterior and middle scaleni may also directly lead to compromise of the brachial plexus and subclavian artery by decreasing the relative space between the two muscles.

Special tests, such as Adson's maneuver, the military position (exaggerated shoulder girdle retraction and depression), and hyperabduction of the shoulder are used to determine the site of entrapment among the three most common sites described previous.[53] Grieve gives a detailed analysis of how cervical spine, shoulder girdle, and upper extremity positional changes during the three classical tests can alter the stresses on the neurovascular bundle. He also discusses the potential for false positive findings.[47] Although these tests may be of diagnostic value, they are of little value in helping one determine which specific dysfunction needs to be treated. The clinician must rely on other components of the examination for this information.

Any joint dysfunction and/or muscle imbalance found in the upper quarter should be treated with the hope of directly or indirectly relieving stress on the brachial plexus and subclavian vessels. An example would be costovertebral joint dysfunction, which results in elevation of the first rib. To relieve the compressive forces on the neurovascular bundle one would have to treat the joint dysfunction, allowing the first rib to resume its normal position. Other joints which could be involved in producing TOS include the sternoclavicular, acromioclavicular, glenohumeral, and the joints of the cervical and thoracic spine.

Muscle imbalances are also commonly found in the pregnant woman presenting with excessive FHP and TOS symptoms. These imbalances may have been one of the factors resulting in the abnormal FHP and/or a result of the development of FHP during pregnancy. Weakness is often found in the shoulder retractors, with associated tightness in the shoulder protractors. Muscle tightness of the cervical spine, including the scaleni and levator scapula, is also commonly present. These muscle imbalances may not allow the woman to assume a more correct, upright posture. This inability to move out of the FHP position produces a more constant stress on the structures involved in TOS and may lead to the onset of symptoms.

A home exercise to stretch cervical spine muscles that may be tight is shown in Figure 2-3. To stretch the left side the patient sits erect in a chair and

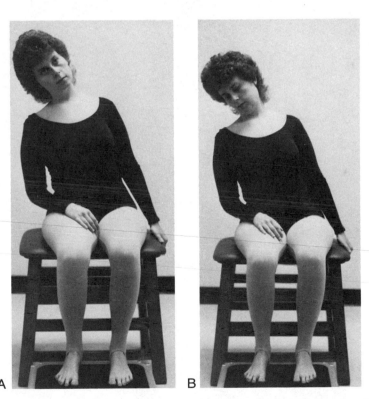

Fig. 2-3. (A) Self-stretch for left sides cervical musculature. (B) Varying degrees of neck rotation can change the focus of the stretch.

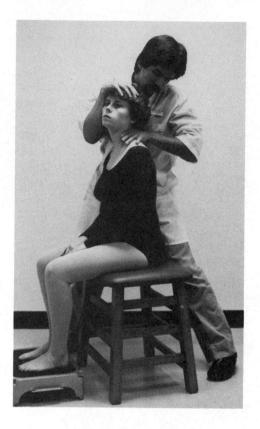

Fig. 2-4. Foraminal closure maneuver for stressing structures within the left intervertebral foramen and weight bearing structures on the left side of the neck.

grasps the left side of the chair with her left hand. The patient side bends her head and neck to the right, then leans her trunk to the right, maintaining a side bent position. The left hand grasping the chair anchors the left shoulder girdle and ribs, allowing for a stretch of the left-sided soft tissue structures. By including cervical rotation to the left or right and incorporating varying degrees of forward bending or backward bending, the stretch can be somewhat localized to a specific region of the cervical spine. This process can be repeated for a stretch of the right-sided structures. Exhaling as the patient stretches will enhance the overall effect of the exercise.

When a patient presents with neck and upper extremity symptoms, one must be aware that the neurologic signs and symptoms often classically attributed to TOS may be of cervical origin. Spinal cord or nerve compression in the cervical spine may result in upper extremity pain, weakness, and altered sensation. A special test, the foraminal closure maneuver (Fig. 2-4), selectively stresses the spinal segment by closing down the ipsilateral intervertebral foramen. If radiating pain and/or neurologic signs are provoked, treatment to relieve the compression forces can be localized to the involved segment. In addition, areas outside the upper quarter may have to be addressed when treating these patients. For example, lumbar spine dysfunction may not allow the patient to assume an appropriate upright standing or sitting posture.

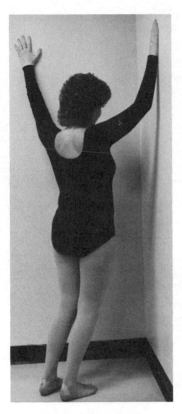
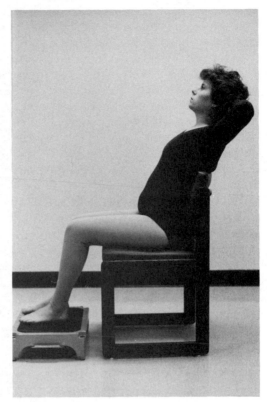

Fig. 2-5. Corner stretch for pectoral muscle groups.

Fig. 2-6. Self-mobilization for backward bending in the thoracic spine.

Compensation in the upper quarter could place abnormal stress on the associated structures, leading to symptoms.

Other conditions besides TOS can be provoked by the postural changes found during pregnancy. The increased thoracic kyphosis compensating for an increased lumbar lordosis and enlarging breasts may place excessive stress on the posterior structures of the thoracic spine. These structures may include muscles, ligaments, facet joints, intervertebral discs, and rib joints. Any pre-existing thoracic dysfunction which is usually aggravated by excessive forward bending may be further irritated by the increase in thoracic kyphosis. To minimize the potential harmful effects of progressive thoracic kyphosis, the clinician must evaluate the thorax for soft tissue imbalances and joint dysfunction. Anterior soft tissue restrictions from tight pectoral muscle groups and abdominal and thoracic scars could prevent the woman from reversing the kyphotic curve to a significant degree. An effective home stretch for anterior soft tissue structures is a modification of the prone press-up described by McKenzie.[41,54] Instead of emphasizing lumbar extension while the pelvis is kept on the floor, the patient should emphasize elevation and anterior expansion of the thorax with the head and neck extended. If the pelvis is kept firmly on the floor, the patient should feel a good stretch anteriorly.

To stretch the pectorals at home, the commonly used corner stretch can be effective (Fig. 2-5). As the woman becomes more pregnant, she may choose to hang on to either side of a doorframe as she stretches the pectorals. The patient may change the hand position by further elevating the arms in order to alter the focus of the stretch on the muscle. Weakness of muscle groups such as the rhomboids, trapezius, and erector spinae could prevent the woman from maintaining a more erect posture if she had the ability to assume one. Strengthening exercises for these muscles could safely be done in sitting, standing, or hands–knees position.

To improve joint mobility of the thoracic spine, a good home exercise for the patient is illustrated in Figure 2-6. With the back of the chair stabilizing the caudal vertebrae, the stretch to the thoracic spine is fairly localized. Having the patient exhale as she stretches into backward bending will enhance the stretch. The patient may position herself to stabilize different vertebrae against the back of the chair by sliding down in the chair, by sitting more erect, or by sitting on pillows. If followed diligently, these and other home exercises, combined with appropriate clinical treatment, may relieve enough stress on the involved upper quarter structures to give the pregnant woman significant relief.

EXAMINATION OF THE LUMBAR SPINE AND PELVIS IN THE OBSTETRIC PATIENT

In evaluating the lumbar spine, pelvis, and lower extremities of the pregnant female, the physical therapist must be able to assess structure and posture, active and passive mobility, muscle balance, position and condition of various tissues, and response to provocation without compromising the mother or the fetus. What follows is a list of evaluation procedures outlined by position as found clinically useful to the author. Suggested modifications for the pregnant patient will be discussed.

I. Standing
  A. Observation and palpation of structure, posture, and position
    1. Compare posture to plumb line ideal[39]
      a. Note position of head and neck
      b. Note position of shoulders and scapula
      c. Note shape of thoracic curve and rib cage
      d. Note presence of scoliotic curve
      e. Note shape of lumbar lordosis
      f. Check for presence of lateral shift[41]
      g. Compare iliac crest heights
      h. Compare posterior superior iliac spine (PSIS) position
      i. Compare anterior superior iliac spine (ASIS) position

        j. Note differences in gluteal bulk and tone

        k. Compare gluteal fold heights

        l. Compare greater trochanter heights

        m. Note position and shape of thighs, knees, lower legs

        n. Note position of feet and ankles

  B. Observation of gait pattern

    1. Check if weight is effectively distributed over center of gravity

    2. Check for presence of Trendelenburg sign

    3. Check for symmetrical hip drop

    4. Check for equal stride length

    5. Look for asymmetries in foot, ankle, knee, on hip function

  C. Active mobility tests

    1. Spine

        a. Backward bending

        b. Side bending

        c. Hip drop[33,43] (Fig. 2-7)

        d. Forward bending

    2. Iliosacral mobility

        a. Forward bend test

        b. March test

  D. Passive Mobility tests

    1. Observe and feel ability of spine to side glide[41] (Fig. 2-8)

  E. Strength tests

    1. Toe up (S1 myotome)

    2. Heel walk (L4 myotome)

    3. One-legged stance (lateral hip musculature)

II. Sitting

  A. Observation and palpation of structure, posture, and position

    1. Note habitual posture assumed

    2. Note positional changes that may have occurred with removal of lower quarter influence

        a. Upper quarter

        b. Scoliotic curve

        c. Thoracic kyphosis

        d. Lumbar lordosis

        e. Iliac crest heights

        f. PSIS position

        g. Compare anteroposterior position of inferior lateral angle (ILA) of sacrum in neutral, full flexion, and extension.[33,40]

        h. Compare anteroposterior position of lumbar and low thoracic transverse processes in neutral, full flexion, and extension[33,40] (Fig. 2-9).

  B. Active mobility

    1. Spine

        a. Forward bending

        b. Backward bending

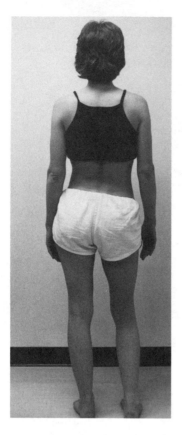

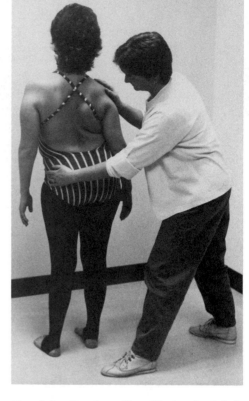

Fig. 2-7. Hip drop test in standing.

Fig. 2-8. Passive side glide to the left in standing.

       c. Rotation with arms crossed over chest
       d. Lateral elongation in sitting (Fig. 2-10A)
    2. Sacral mobility
       a. Forward bending test
C. Passive mobility
    1. Spinal mobility
       a. Combined rotation and side bending with flexion[33]
       b. Combined rotation and side bending with extension[33]
       c. Side bending in neutral
D. Palpation for tissue tension changes
    1. Palpate lateral to spinous processes for increased tension in the small rotators
    2. Look and feel for edema, trophic changes, tenderness
E. Neurologic Examination
    1. Deep tendon reflexes

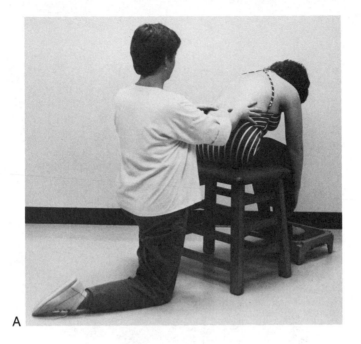

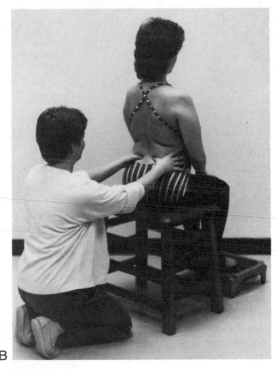

Fig. 2-9. (A) Vertebral position testing with spine in flexion. **(B)** Vertebral position testing with spine in extension.

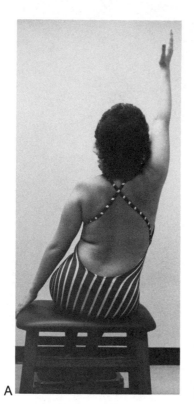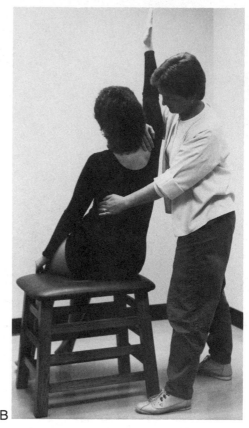

Fig. 2-10. **(A)** Elongation of the spine to the right in sitting. **(B)** Sitting elongation with assist.

         a. Ankle jerk
         b. Knee jerk
      2. Strength tests
         a. Psoas (L1–2)
         b. Quadriceps (L3–4)
         c. Ankle dorsiflexors (L4)
         d. Extensor hallucis longus (L5)
         e. Peroneals (L5)
         f. Hamstrings (L5–S1)
III. Supine
    A. Observation and palpation of structure and position
      1. Observe lower extremity resting positions
      2. Observe trunk and pelvis position in lying
      3. Compare ASIS positions
      4. Check for unleveling and tenderness of the pubic symphysis
      5. Supine to sit test

   B. Active mobility
      1. Hips
      2. Knees
      3. Ankles
   C. Passive mobility
      1. Endfeel test for passive hip, knee, ankle range of motion
      2. Muscle length tests
         a. Hamstrings
         b. Hip adductors
         c. Piriformis
         d. Hip flexors (Thomas test position[37])
            1. Check iliotibial band, internal/external rotators, abductors, rectus femoris in Thomas test position
         e. Gastroc-soleus
      3. Provocation tests
         a. Hip joint
            1. Faber test (flexion, abduction, external rotation)
            2. Scouring
         b. Lumbar flexion with both knees to chest with repetitions
   D. Neurologic Examination
      1. Resistive tests
         a. Hip flexors (L2)
         b. Quadriceps (L3)
         c. Anterior tibialis (L4)
         d. Extensor hallucis longus (L5)
      2. Sensory Examination
      3. Straight leg raise
         a. Dural stretch
   E. Strength tests
      1. Abdominals
         a. Upper abdominal curls
         b. Leg slides with back flat
      2. Functional ability to "bridge"
   F. Evaluation of transverse fascial planes[49]
IV. Sidelying
   A. Passive mobility testing
      1. Lumbar side bending with flexion or in neutral
      2. Rocking ilium by abduction/adduction of the flexed hip
   B. Strength tests
      1. Hip abductors
         a. Resistive
         b. Firing patterns[55]
V. Prone
   A. Observation and palpation of structure and position
      1. Compare iliac crest position
      2. Compare PSIS position

   3. Compare ischial tuberosity position
   4. Compare anteroposterior and inferior-superior positions of ILAs of sacrum in neutral and in extension (prone prop)[33,40,42]
   5. Compare anteroposterior positions of low thoracic and lumbar transverse processes in neutral and extension (prone prop)[33,40,42]
   6. Check leg lengths at heel
B. Palpation for condition
   1. Tenderness
      a. Lateral sacrum and coccyx
      b. Lumbar spinous processes
      c. Soft tissues
   2. Swelling
      a. Specific lumbar segments
      b. Local swelling at sacrum
   3. Muscle tone
      a. Guarding or hypertonic
      b. Atrophy
   4. Skin condition
   5. Tension in the sacrotuberous ligament
C. Active mobility
   1. Prone press-ups[41]
      a. As provocation test
      b. As mobility test
   1. Hip extension
      a. Observe firing pattern[55]
      b. Resisted
D. Passive mobility
   1. Spine
      a. Rotation through lower extremities with spine in neutral or extension[38,42]
      b. Oscillatory mobility tests[30]
         1. Unilateral on transverse processes
         2. Transverse pressures on spinous processes
         3. Central pressure on spinous processes
   2. Sacral mobility
      a. Extension of sacral base by posteroanterior pressure on opposite ILA, one at a time
      b. Flexion of sacral base by direct pressure at sulcus, one at a time
      c. Palpation of both sacral bases as the patient does press-ups
   3. Hips
      a. Passive external rotation and internal rotation with knees flexed
      b. Rectus femoris length with opposite leg flexed over the edge of the table[45] (Fig. 2-11)
E. Strength tests
   1. Gluteus maximus
   2. Hamstrings

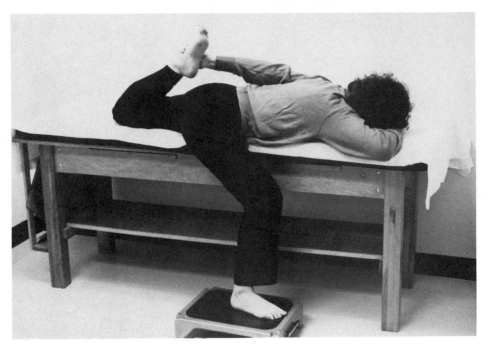

Fig. 2-11. Test and/or stretch for left rectus femoris muscle to be used if patient can still tolerate prone lying.

VI. All fours (hands-knees)
  A. Observation and palpation of structure and position
    1. Palpate position of transverse processes in neutral, flexion, and extension (Fig. 2-12)
    2. Have patient rock forward and back while in extension; observe levels of prominent transverse processes as motion occurs at each segment from thoracolumbar junction through lumbosacral junction
    3. Observe elongation of spine with side to side weight shift
    4. Observe ability of both sacral bases to extend as the patient sits back in the "prayer stretch" position

Testing in the Standing Position

Observation and palpation can begin in the standing position. The therapist should note where the pregnant woman is carrying her weight to see if she has adapted her posture to efficiently accommodate. When observing the gait pattern, signs of joint instability or muscle weakness should be noted.

Standing active mobility tests for the spine should demonstrate smoothness of curve and symmetrical recruitment. Check for flat spots indicating

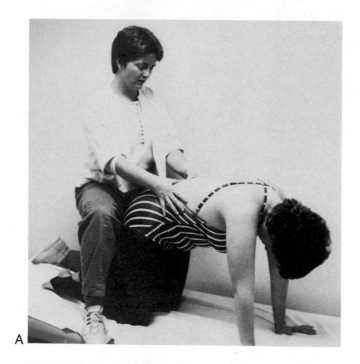

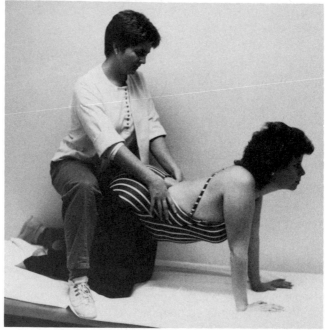

Fig. 2-12. **(A)** Palpation for vertebral position with spine in flexion. **(B)** Palpation for vertebral position with spine in extension.

restriction, fulcrums, or shifts indicating possible instability. Look for deviations from the midline and make note of juddering or hitching in the range.

The hip drop test in standing gives information regarding side bending mobility in the lumbosacral region. The therapist asks the patient to stand with her weight on both feet. She is instructed to keep one knee straight while allowing the other knee to bend and drop the hip (Fig. 2-7). The amount of excursion is compared side to side as the side bending curve is observed in the low lumbar area.[33]

Mobility of the ilium on the sacrum is assessed with the standing forward bend test and the march test. The therapist places the thumbs under the patient's PSISs and compares motion as the patient bends forward. After an initial slack time, both PSIS should move simultaneously and with equal excursion. Early or further excursion of one PSIS may indicate restricted mobility of the ilium on that side or may demonstrate that the hamstrings of the opposite leg are tight. Further information is gained as the patient marches in place with the therapist's thumbs under the PSIS. Amounts of posterior ilial rotation can be compared side to side during hip flexion, while amounts of anterior ilial rotation can be compared during stance phase.

Passive side gliding of the spine to the right in standing is tested by pressing down and toward the right on the left shoulder while simultaneously pressing the right hip toward the left (Fig. 2-8). This is then compared to the side gliding in standing to the left.

Testing in the Sitting Position

Observation of structure and posture as well as active mobility tests are also performed in sitting in order to assess what influence the lower quarter may have had in standing. Rotation of the spine is more easily observed in sitting since the pelvis and hips are stabilized. One can get a sense of the patient's ability to side bend in both directions by observing lateral elongation of the spine with rocking side to side in sitting (Fig. 2-10A).

The forward bend test in sitting is a screening test for sacral mobility. The physical therapist places the thumbs under the PSISs as the patient bends forward from the sitting position. Amounts of PSIS excursion are compared at the end range. Further excursion of one PSIS may indicate restriction of sacral base mobility on that side.[33]

The sitting position is very useful for assessing the pregnant woman's passive spinal mobility, especially in combined motions such as rotation and side bending with extension. Palpation of tissue tension increase in the small rotator muscles lateral to the spinous processes may indicate to the examiner that joint dysfunction exists at that level. One also palpates bony and soft tissue structures for edema, trophic changes, and tenderness. The neurologic examination can be continued in sitting by testing ankle and knee jerk reflexes and performing some of the myotome strength tests.

Supine Testing

Women in the second and third trimesters of pregnancy should not be kept in the supine position for extended periods of time. Supine testing should be broken into short intervals. Observation and palpation of bony and soft tissue structures are performed in the supine position; the examiner should make sure to compare the heights of the two sides of the pubic symphysis. The supine-to-sit test is a screening test for pelvic joint dysfunction. The therapist compares the supine and long-sitting leg lengths at the medial malleoli. A change from one position to the other may indicate asymmetrical iliac position. Active and passive mobility tests for the hips, knees, and ankles are easily conducted in the supine position. Strength and length of some of the muscles of the hips, trunk, and pelvis are also tested in supine. The lumbar spine can be tested for provocation in flexion by pulling the knees to chest, and hip provocation tests can also be carried out.

Evaluation of transverse fascial plane mobility is performed in the supine position at the pelvic and thoracic diaphragms, the thoracic inlet, and the suboccipital region. If the patient is unable to lie supine, this can also be done in standing, sitting, or sidelying.[49] Fascial restriction may proliferate joint and soft tissue dysfunction.

Testing in Sidelying, Pronelying, and Hands-Knees

Sidelying can be used as an alternative evaluation position for observation and palpation, but care should be taken to maintain the normal alignment of the spine in the midsagittal plane. Sidelying is a comfortable and appropriate position for testing certain passive lumbar motions and assessing function of the hip abductor muscles.

Prone is a position usually avoided after the first trimester. The patient in her first trimester could still tolerate pronelying with one leg flexed over the edge of the table; this allows easy assessment of rectus femoris length while the spine is stabilized (Fig. 2-11). Strength tests for gluteus maximus and observation of hip extensor firing patterns are most easily performed with the patient lying prone.[55] During the latter stages of pregnancy much of the information gleaned from prone testing can be determined in sitting or in the all-fours or hands-knees position.

The hands-knees position is one of relative ease for most pregnant women and is a good position for assessing spinal flexion and extension. In this position the hip flexors are slack, and weight bearing through the spine itself is reduced. One should remember that soft tissue imbalances or a difference in femur length may affect pelvis and lumbar position in hands-knees.

TREATMENT OF THE LUMBAR SPINE AND PELVIS IN THE OBSTETRIC PATIENT

Treatment of lumbar spine, pelvis, and lower quarter dysfunction in the pregnant population is the same as for the nonpregnant population except that the therapist must take precautions with positioning the patient and must at all times be aware of the increased ligamentous laxity and relative vulnerability of the connective tissues due to the effects of relaxin. Therapists are cautioned to avoid heavy traction techniques[56] and vigorous manipulations[6] with pregnant patients. Generally, it is good to start with the most gentle treatment techniques available and proceed carefully with more aggressive techniques only if necessary. Whenever possible, the patient should be instructed in self-treatment methods.

Therapists should be aware of the general rationale for treatment of disc derangement, spondylolisthesis, thoracic, lumbar, hip and pelvic joint dysfunctions, and muscle imbalances. Knowledge of orthotic treatment for abnormally functioning feet and ankles is also of great help, as poor foot alignment may affect the mechanics of the entire lower kinetic chain and spine.

Conditions that are neurologically threatening should receive top management priority. If a pregnant woman presents with signs of nerve root compression, such as loss of motor strength, reflexes, or objective sensory loss, the therapist must consider the possibility of disc derangement or herniation, spondylolisthesis, or lateral stenosis. Because radiologic diagnosis is generally avoided during pregnancy, one must rely on clinical presentation. As surgery for spinal problems is rarely performed during pregnancy except in cases of neurologic emergency,[5,6] the therapist's task is to help the patient achieve greater comfort and hopefully decrease the patient's signs of neurologic compromise. This initially entails finding the resting positions that most effectively decrease the symptoms. As the patient improves, attempts should be made to increase mobility and function without re-exacerbating the condition.

Disc Derangement

Robin McKenzie presents a clinically effective self-management regime for disc derangement in his books, *The Lumbar Spine: Mechanical Diagnosis and Therapy*[39] and *Treat Your Own Back*.[54] If a pregnant woman presents with low back pain and/or lower extremity pain with loss of lumbar lordosis and a lateral shift, attempts should be made to regain midline stance and normal spinal extension. Self shift correction can be done in standing position (Fig. 2-13), and improvement of backward bending can be achieved from the hands-knees position or in standing, although prone press-ups are the first method of choice if the patient is in her first trimester and can still tolerate lying

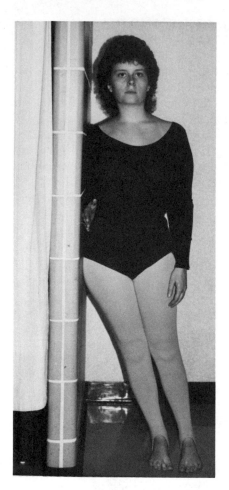

Fig. 2-13. Self-correction of right lateral shift.

prone. If the patient is unable to achieve self-correction, the therapist may find with passive and positional testing that one or more spinal segments are in dysfunction and may require mobilization. Muscle energy mobilization techniques for the spine[33,42,43] may be used gently and effectively with pregnant women in either sidelying or sitting positions.

Spondylolisthesis

Spondylolisthesis is a pre-existing condition which may worsen with pregnancy as the patient's weight increases low and anterior.[3] With isthmic spondylolisthesis, anterior slippage of the superior vertebral body on the inferior one occurs due to a fracture of the pars interarticularis, leaving the posterior elements behind. This most often occurs at the L5–S1 level. A vertebra may also slip forward on the one below if the facet joints are extremely eroded, causing widening of the facet joint spaces and laxity of the capsules. This degenerative spondylolisthesis most commonly occurs at L4-L5, where the facets are more sagittally oriented and are less able to structurally prevent the forward slip.[9] The pregnant woman with spondylolisthesis must be instructed in effective posterior pelvic tilt maneuvers. This almost always requires first stretching out the iliopsoas and rectus femoris muscles to decrease the anterior pull on the pelvis and lumbar spine. (Recommended stretching methods are delineated below in the section on muscle imbalances.) Spondylolisthesis is frequently accompanied by sacroiliac joint dysfunction,[9] and evaluation and treatment for this and other possible lumbar and thoracic joint and soft tissue dysfunctions should be included in management.

Joint and Soft Tissue Dysfunction

Many patients can effectively self-treat joint and soft tissue dysfunction with a carefully designed exercise program. Self-mobilizing exercises are particularly useful during pregnancy since the patient may be vulnerable to injury from more aggressive techniques.

The hands-knees position is a particularly good exercise position for pregnant women. It allows the weight of the uterus to fall forward out of the pelvic cavity, relieving pressure on the blood vessels and nerves that lie anterior to the spine. Rhythmic pelvic rocking exercises (cat backs) not only mobilize the spine in flexion and extension but also provide mild toning activity for the abdominals and buttocks while allowing improved circulation and decreased congestion in the pelvis, buttocks, and upper thighs.[57] The spinal mobility gained by doing this exercise can be made more specific to various parts of the spine by shifting the weight forward or back. The more forward one shifts, the more local the exercise becomes for the lumbosacral region; as one shifts further back, more mobility will occur in the area of the thoracolumbar junction. If one places the hands closer to the knees or rests on the forearms rather than the hands, more movement can be achieved in the thoracic spine and interscapular region.

The hands-knees position can also be used to improve side bending by using a hip-hiking or "tail-wagging" motion. Side bending in hands-knees can be done with the spine in neutral, but can also be performed in the flexed or extended positions to promote combined motions. The fulcrum of motion can be varied with this exercise by either shifting the weight forward or backward, as previously described.

Side bending mobility can also be improved by sitting elongation (Fig. 2-10A). As the patient shifts her weight onto the right buttock, she lifts the left buttock while simultaneously stretching upward with the right arm. Not only will this improve movement patterns in the spine, but it will allow the pregnant woman relief of the compressed feeling that occurs in the lower rib cage as the baby grows larger. The therapist may provide manual direction with this exercise either to specify the fulcrum of movement or to encourage further range (Fig. 2-10B).

The Lumbar Spine and Pelvis

Osteopathic literature recommends that treatment of the lumbar spine and pelvis usually be done in a specific order; that is, first the spine, then the pubis, the sacrum, and lastly the ilia.[33] Once the functioning of the spine itself has been improved by either postural correction, self-mobilizing exercises, or specific mobilization techniques, the other areas should be addressed and treated.

Some degree of pubic separation is normal for many pregnant women, but it may become symptomatic if the separation is extreme or if further stress from trauma is placed on the already vulnerable joint.[2,3,5,11,15,16] Support can be achieved by the use of a pelvic belt especially designed for pregnant women. The support commonly used with success by the author was designed by Jim Porterfield, P.T., and is available through I.E.M. Products (Fig. 2-14). It provides some stability for the lumbosacral junction and the sacroiliac joints as well as the pubic symphysis.[48] Should unleveling of the pubic symphysis occur, the patient will usually present with groin and adductor pain. The difference in pubic levels will be palpated at the pubic symphysis, and the forward bending test in standing position will be positive. The standing march test with thumbs on the PSISs helps determine the dysfunctional side, as a superior or inferior pubis will usually create apparent movement dysfunction of the corresponding iliosacral joint. Muscle energy techniques using the hip adductors may be used to correct a superior pube. An inferior pube is most effectively treated by the use of gentle direct pressure to the ischial tuberosity and the anterior ilium.[33,43] Resistance to the hip extensor muscles may facilitate this mobilization.

Joint dysfunction or disc derangement in the lumbar spine is often accompanied by sacral dysfunction. If after treating the lumbar spine and pubis the therapist still finds positional and mobility tests at the sacrum to be abnormal, improvement may be achieved by using direct mobilization techniques or muscle energy techniques in sidelying, sitting, supine, or prone positions. Detailed description of sacral correction techniques using chiefly the piriformis muscle and the lumbar paravertebrals are given in Mitchell, Moran, and Pruzo's book, *An Evaluation and Treatment Manual of Osteopathic Muscle Energy Procedures.*[33] A thorough understanding of the clinical biomechanics of sacral mobility is necessary to properly evaluate and treat the sacroiliac joints, as many apparent positional and mobility problems of the ilia are actually secondary to sacral problems. A therapist who treats only ilial dysfunction without evaluating and treating the lumbar spine, pubis, and sacrum may actually be creating more problems in the long term.

Many ilial problems are created or proliferated by muscle imbalances. In all patients but especially in pregnant women whose ligamentous structures are

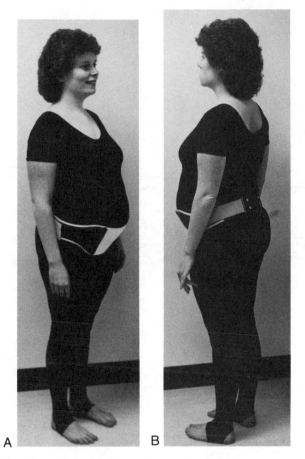

Fig. 2-14. (A,B) Maternity lumbopelvic support belt available through IEM products.

so vulnerable to injury, mobilization for an apparent iliac dysfunction should be preceded by stretching of shortened muscles and strengthening of weakened muscles. Should tests for ilial positional faults and mobility dysfunction continue to be positive even after treating the surrounding joints and soft tissues, then gentle mobilization procedures should be employed.

The ilium may be restricted in anterior or posterior rotation, inflare or outflare, or a combination of these. Upslips and downslips of the ilium may occur with trauma. Many times a pregnant woman may effectively correct an anteriorly or posteriorly rotated ilium simply by positioning herself to encourage movement in the desired direction (Fig. 2-15). Should this not achieve sufficient correction, the next method of choice would be muscle energy techniques.[33] Contractions of hip flexors, rectus femoris, or adductors with the distal attachment fixed can be used to bring the ilium anterior, while contrac-

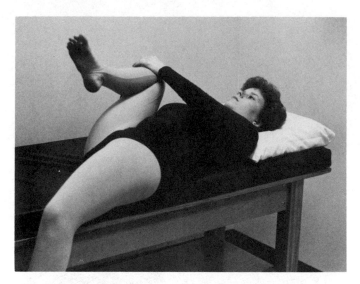

Fig. 2-15.   Self-correction of ilial rotation by positioning.

tion of hamstrings or gluteus maximus will bring the ilium posterior. Stabilization of the opposite ilium and lumbar spine are essential for achieving effective mobilization.[33,42,43] More aggressive mobilization is rarely necessary for pregnant women, but if one finds the use of direct techniques unavoidable, they should be employed gently and slowly. High velocity thrust techniques should be avoided.[6]

Soft Tissue Imbalances

Muscle imbalances frequently found in the area of the lumbar spine, hips, and pelvis involve shortening of the iliacus, psoas, rectus femoris, piriformis, thoracolumbar junction and upper lumbar paravertebrals, hamstrings, adductors, tensor fascia latae, and gastroc-soleus, usually accompanied by weakness of the abdominals, gluteus maximus, gluteus medius, low lumbar paravertebrals, and sometimes the quadriceps[37,55]. Imbalance of the soft tissues can create and proliferate joint dysfunctions and should be treated concurrently with mobilization techniques. Various methods employed by physical therapists that may help to decrease soft tissue restrictions include myofascial release, craniosacral therapy,[49] and deep connective tissue massage.[58] Dr. John Upledger, D.O., states that craniosacral therapy and myofascial release are very appropriate means for treating pregnant women, as they are both gentle and effective (personal communication, West Palm Beach Fla., 1986). Patients should be instructed in stretching and strengthening methods if they can tolerate exercise.

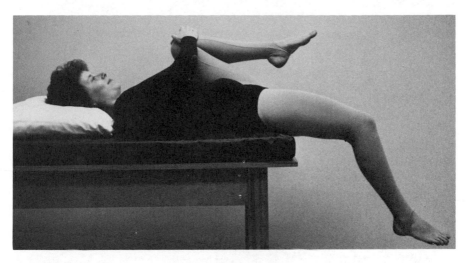

Fig. 2-16.   Stretch of the right hip flexor muscles in the Thomas test position.

Stretching Exercises

Effective stretching demands proper stabilization, and positioning should also ensure that the spine is in a protected position. In her first trimester of pregnancy, a woman can use the familiar Thomas test position to stretch her iliopsoas. As she lies supine with her hips at the edge of the table, one knee is held firmly to the chest while the other leg hangs over the edge. Contracting the buttocks of the down leg will assist in the stretch (Fig. 2-16). If the thigh is held down, flexing the knee will add a gentle stretch to the rectus femoris. As the pregnancy progresses, the half kneel position is more favorable for iliopsoas stretching. The woman kneels on the side to be stretched. It is essential that she be able to hold a strong posterior tilt of the pelvis during the stretch, as slight flexion of the lumbar spine must be maintained. She keeps her hand on the buttocks of the stretching side and taps to facilitate the gluteal contraction that brings about the stretch of the hip flexors as she pulls forward with the opposite leg (Fig. 2-17). If a patient is able to maintain this position well, she can add a stretch to the rectus femoris by flexing the knee that is on the ground and grasping the ankle. She must continue to hold a strong posterior pelvic tilt.[58]

Standing tensor fasciae latae stretches can probably be tolerated throughout pregnancy. The woman stands so that the side to be stretched is toward the wall. While leaning with her hand or forearm against the wall, she crosses the leg to be stretched behind her. Keeping her trunk straight, she then leans her hip toward the wall, allowing the front knee to bend (Fig. 2-18). The position should be maintained for at least 20 to 30 seconds. If necessary, the therapist can help the patient with tensor fasciae latae stretches from the Thomas test position in supine by adducting the hip and keeping the tibia internally rotated as the hip is extended.

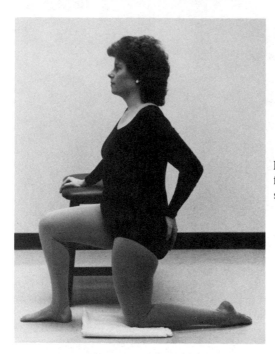

Fig. 2-17. Stretch of the left hip flexor muscles in the half-kneel position.

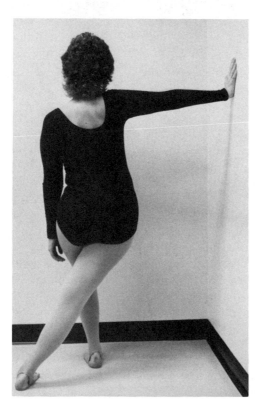

Fig. 2-18. Stretch for the right tensor fascia latae muscle in standing.

The piriformis can be stretched in sitting or supine by flexing, adducting, and internally rotating the hip while keeping the spine straight and the pelvis level (Fig. 2-19). If done in supine lying, the opposite leg should be anchored by tightening the quadriceps and holding the leg down flat.

Hamstring stretches in the supine position can be achieved by flexing the hip 90 degrees, grasping the distal thigh with both hands, and attempting to straighten the knee while anchoring the opposite leg by holding it flat with the quadriceps tightened (Fig. 2-20). If supine lying is not favorable, a variety of yoga exercises in the Iyengar style[59-61] can be used to stretch the hamstrings while paying attention to spinal stability and alignment. One possibility is the wall stretch (Fig. 2-21), done by keeping the quadriceps tight and the kneecaps pulled up as the spine is actively elongated by pushing the ischial tuberosities up and back as the hands push away from the wall. *Stretch and Relax*, by Tobias and Stewart, is a good pictorial reference for other Iyengar-style yoga stretches; it has sections on pregnancy and postpartum.[61]

Adductors can be gently stretched in an erect sitting position with the soles of the feet placed together or while lying supine and maintaining a pelvic tilt. The patient may find it easier to let go of the adductors gradually by allowing

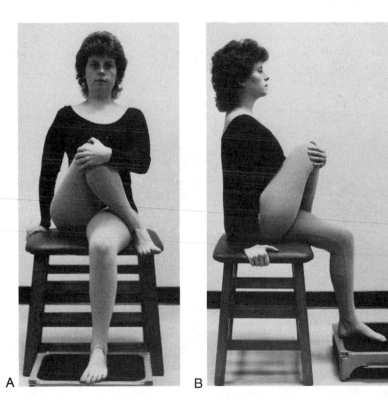

A   B

Fig. 2-19. (A,B) Stretch for the right piriformis muscle in sitting.

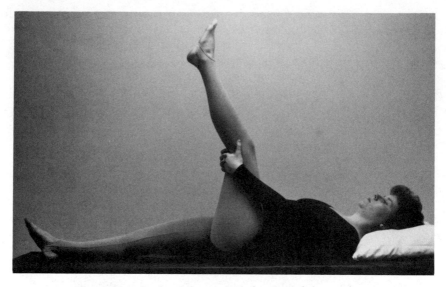

Fig. 2-20.   Supine lying stretch for the left hamstring.

the thighs to be gently supported by pillows (Fig. 2-22). Thoracolumbar junction and upper lumbar paravertebrals can be stretched in the prayer stretch position, in which the woman sinks back towards the heels from the hands-knees position. As she becomes more pregnant, she may need to separate the knees to make room for the uterus.

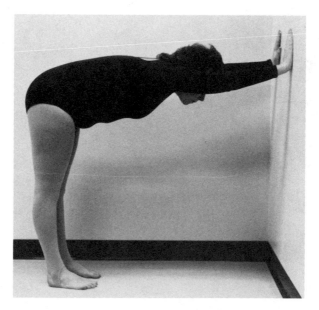

Fig. 2-21.   Wall stretch for bilateral hamstrings with attempted spine elongation.

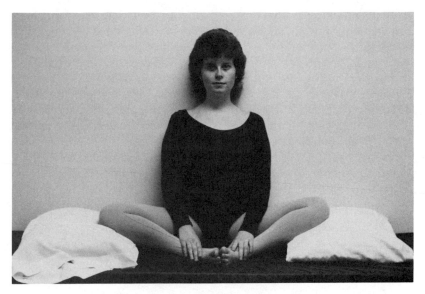

Fig. 2-22.   Gradual bilateral adductor stretch with spine supported.

Standing calf stretches should be part of the woman's exercise routine since cramps in the gastroc-soleus group are so common during pregnancy.[62] Standing stretches in the lunge position can usually be performed throughout pregnancy, but passive stretch of the posterior calf muscles can be provided by a partner who dorsiflexes the ankle while holding the knee in extension as the patient sits or lies supine.

Strengthening Exercises

Strengthening exercises for the gluteus maximus and medius should be performed throughout the pregnancy in order to maintain support for the increasingly vulnerable joints of the pelvis. Supine bridging exercises, either with legs extended and supported on a low stool or with hips and knees bent and feet flat on the floor, are a good way to exercise the buttocks without placing stress on the spine. The feet and knees should be kept hip width apart as the woman performs a posterior pelvic tilt and then raises the buttocks off the surface until the trunk is in line with the knees and shoulders. Hip extension may be performed from the hands-knees position for gluteus maximus strengthening, but the woman should take care to maintain a neutral position of the spine so as not to proliferate abnormal hip extensor firing patterns and place a strain on the lumbar spine.

Gluteus medius strengthening from the hands-knees position is very effective for the pregnant woman. She starts in a stable position with hands under the shoulders and knees under the hips. As she maintains her pelvic tilt, she sinks diagonally toward one hip as if moving toward a side-sitting position. She stops the motion when she is about halfway to the floor. When she begins to feel contraction in the area of the gluteus medius, she should then move partway back up toward her starting position. She can then move back into her hip-sink position and repeat the procedure several times before returning to neutral. She can then repeat the process, only moving toward the opposite hip.

The appropriateness of certain abdominal strengthening exercises during pregnancy is somewhat controversial (see the section on etiology of diastasis recti in Ch. 3). Probably the safest abdominal exercises for a pregnant woman to do are pelvic tilts in the hands-knees position (cat backs) and supine leg slides while maintaining a strong pelvic tilt.[62] Pregnant women should be cautioned not to remain in the supine position for extended periods of time, and exercises while lying supine should be interspersed between exercises in other positions.

SUMMARY

The purpose of this chapter has been to present an evaluation and treatment rationale for musculoskeletal problems that may arise during pregnancy. It is meant to give the physical therapist an idea of the background necessary for understanding this unique patient population. An OB/GYN physical therapist should seek further education in orthopedic PT in order to provide the pregnant woman with the best conservative care possible. Numerous texts which may be helpful have been referenced in this chapter, and many short courses in musculoskeletal evaluation and treatment are currently available to the postgraduate PT. Another valuable resource for information is the increasing number of graduate programs in orthopedic physical therapy.

A need exists for further documentation and research as to the efficacy and reliability of physical therapy assessment and treatment procedures, particularly in the area of observation and palpation. As physical therapists continue to assess and treat movement dysfunction, they should strive for the best and most careful evaluation and treatment procedures possible.

ACKNOWLEDGMENTS

We wish to thank Sandy Klein, Jill Boissonnault, M.S., P.T., and Melissa Shirriff, P.T., for their assistance as photographic models. We also thank our photographer, Donald Darling, M.S., P.T.

REFERENCES

1. Bushnell LF: The postural pains of pregnancy. Part I, Parietal neuralgia of pregnancy. Western Journal of Surgery, Obstetrics and Gynecology, March:123, 1949

2. Romen Y, Artal R: Physiological and endocrine adjustments to pregnancy. p. 59. In Artal R, Wiswell RA (eds): Exercise in Pregnancy. Williams & Wilkins, Baltimore, 1986

3. Spankus JD: The cause and treatment of low back pain during pregnancy. Wisconsin Med J 64:303, 1965

4. Fries EC, Hellebrandt FA: The influence of pregnancy on the location of the center of gravity, postural stability, and body alignment. Am J Obstet and Gyn 46:374, 1943

5. Epstein JA, Benton J, Browder J, et al: Treatment of low back pain and sciatic syndromes during pregnancy. New York State J Med May:1757, 1959

6. Cherry SH, Berkowitz RL, Kase NG (eds): Rovinsky and Guttmacher's Medical, Surgical, and Gynecologic Complications of Pregnancy. 3rd Ed. Williams & Wilkins, Baltimore, 1985

7. Rhodes P: Orthopaedic conditions associated with childbearing. Practitioners 181:304, 1958

8. Ray CD: Percutaneous radiofrequency facet nerve blocks: treatment of the mechanical low back syndrome. Radionics Procedure Techniques Series, 1982

9. Kirkaldy-Willis WH: Managing Low Back Pain. Churchill Livingstone, New York, 1983

10. Darnell MW: A proposed chronology of events for forward head posture. J Craniomandibular Practice 1:49, 1983

11. deSwiet M: The Respiratory System. p 79. In Hytten F and Chamberlain G (eds): Clinical Physiology in Obstetrics. CV Mosby, St. Louis, 1980

12. Berezin D: Pelvic insufficiency during pregnancy and after parturition. Acta Obstet Gyn Scand, 33: suppl. 3, 1954

13. Weiss G: Relaxin. Ann Rev Physiol 46:43, 1984

14. O'Byrne EM, Carriere BT, Sorensen L, et al: Plasma immunoreactive relaxin levels in pregnant and non pregnant women. J Clin Endocrinology and Metab 47:1106, 1978

15. Thorp DJ, Fray WE: The pelvic joints during pregnancy and labor. JAMA Sept:1162, 1938

16. Boland BG: Separation of symphysis pubis. N Engl J Med 208:431, 1933

17. Young J: Relaxation of the pelvic joints in pregnancy: pelvic arthropathy of pregnancy. J Obstet and Gyn of Br Empire 47:493, 1940

18. Friedman MJ: Orthopaedic problems in pregnancy. p. 215. In Artal R, Wiswell RA (eds): Exercise in Pregnancy. Williams & Wilkins, Baltimore, 1986

19. O'Connell JEA: Lumber disc protrusions in pregnancy. J Neurol Neurosurg Psychiatry 23:138, 1960

20. Kelsey J, Greenberg R, Hardy R, et al: Pregnancy and the syndrome of herniated lumbar intervertebral disc: an epidemiological study. Yale J Biol Med 48:361, 1975

21. White AA, Panjabi MM: Clinical Biomechanics of the Spine. JB Lippincott, Philadelphia, 1978

22. Nachemson A: Lumbar intradiscal pressure. p. 347. In Jayson M (ed): The Lumbar Spine and Back Pain. 2nd Ed. Pitman Medical, Turnbridge Wells, 1980

23. Kopell HP, Thompson W: Peripheral Entrapment Neuropathies. Robert E. Krieger Pub Co, Huntington, 1976

24. Position Paper for the Section on Obstetrics and Gynecology. Bulletin of OB GYN Section, APTA, 8:1, 1984

25. Pritchard J, MacDonald P, Grant N: William's Obstetrics. 17th Ed. Appleton-Century-Crofts, E. Norwalk, 1985

26. Kerr M, Scott D, Samuel E: Studies of inferior vena cava in late pregnancy. Br Med J 1:532, 1964

27. Kerr M: The mechanical effects of the gravid uterus in late pregnancy. J Obs Gyn Br Comm 72:513, 1965
28. Isselbacher K, Adams R, Braumwalk E, et al: Harrison's Principles of Internal Medicine. McGraw-Hill, New York, 1980
29. Cyriax J: Textbook of Orthopaedic Medicine. Vol I. 8th Ed. Bailliere Tindall, London, 1980
30. Maitland GD: Vertebral Manipulation. 5th Ed. Butterworth, London, 1986
31. McGuire E (ed): Urinary Incontinence. Grune & Stratton, New York, 1981
32. Stoddard A: Manual of Osteopathic Practice. 2nd Ed. Hutchinson, London, 1983
33. Mitchell FL, Moran PS, Pruzzo NA: An Evaluation and Treatment Manual of Osteopathic Muscle Energy Procedures. Mitchell, Moran, and Pruzzo Assoc, Valley Park, MO 1979
34. Gonella C, Paris S, Kutner M: Reliability in evaluating passive intervertebral motion. Phy Th 62:436, 1982
35. Nyberg RE: Role of physical therapists in spinal manipulation. p. 22. In Basmajian JV (ed): Manipulation, Traction and Massage. Williams & Wilkins, Baltimore, 1985
36. Kendall F, McCreary E: Muscles Testing and Function. 3rd Ed. Williams & Wilkins, Baltimore, 1983
37. Janda V: Muscles, central nervous motor regulation and back problems. p. 27. In Korr I (ed): The Neurophysiological Mechanisms in Manipulative Therapy. Plenum Press, New York, 1978
38. Paris SV: Course Notes . . . The Spine. Institute Press, Atlanta, 1979
39. Kendall HO, Kendall FP, Boynton DA: Posture and Pain. Robert E. Krieger Pub Co, Huntington, 1952
40. Greerman PE: Restricted vertebral motion. Michigan Osteopathic J March:31, 1983
41. McKenzie RA: The Lumbar Spine: Mechanical Diagnosis and Therapy. Spinal Publications, Waikanae, NZ, 1983
42. Lee D, Walsh M: A Workbook of Manual Techniques for the Vertebral Column and Pelvic Girdle. Nascent Publishing, 1985
43. Bourdillon JF: Spinal Manipulation. 3rd Ed. Appleton-Century Crofts, New York, 1982
44. Evjenth O, Hamberg J: Muscle Stretching in Manual Therapy. Vol. II. The Spinal Column and the Temporo-Mandibular Joint. Alfta Rehab, Alfta, Sweden, 1984
45. Evjenth O, Hamberg J: Muscle Stretching in Manual Therapy. Vol. I. The Extremities. Alfta Rehab, Alfta, Sweden, 1984
46. Stoddard A: Manual of Osteopathic Technique. 3rd Ed. Hutchinson, London, 1980
47. Grieve G: Common Vertebral Joint Problems. Churchill Livingstone, Edinburgh, 1981
48. Porterfield JA: The sacroiliac joint. p. 550. In Gould JA, Davies GJ (eds): Orthopaedic and Sports Physical Therapy. Vol. II. CV Mosby, St. Louis, 1985
49. Upledger JE, Vredevooqd JD: Craniosacral Therapy. Eastland Press, Chicago, 1983
50. Williams PL, Warwick R (eds): Gray's Anatomy. 36th Ed. WB Saunders, Philadelphia, 1980
51. Massey E, Cefalo R: Neuropathies of pregnancy. Obs and Gyn Survey 34:489, 1979
52. Anderson JE (ed): Grant's Atlas of Anatomy. 8th Ed. Williams & Wilkins, Baltimore, 1983
53. Lord JW, Rosait LM: Thoracic outlet syndromes. p. 3. In Roberts RH (ed): CIBA 23:2. CIBA Pharmaceutical Company, Summit, NJ, 1971
54. McKenzie RA: Treat Your Own Back. Spinal Publications, Lower Hutt, NZ, 1985

55. Lewit K: Manipulative Therapy in Rehabilitation of the Locomotor System. Butterworth, London, 1985
56. Hinterbuchner C: Traction. p. 191. In Basmajian JV (ed): Manipulation, Traction and Massage. 3rd Ed. Williams & Wilkins, Baltimore, 1985
57. Hartman RE: Exercises for True Natural Childbirth. Harper & Row, New York, 1975
58. Chaitow L: Neuromuscular Technique, A Practitioner's Guide to Soft Tissue Manipulation. Thorsons Publishers Ltd, Wellingborough, 1980
59. Iyengar BKS: Light on Yoga. Schocken Books, New York, 1979
60. Couch J: Runner's World Yoga Book. Anderson World Inc, Mountain View, CA, 1979
61. Tobias M, Stewart M: Stretch and Relax. The Body Press, Tuscon, 1985
62. Noble E: Essential Exercises for the Childbearing Year. Houghton-Mifflin, Boston 1976

3 | Diastasis Recti

Jill Schiff Boissonnault
Rhonda K. Kotarinos

Until recently, diastasis recti received little attention from the medical community in the United States. The recent surge of interest in diastasis recti in this country is primarily due to Elizabeth Noble's discussion of the subject in her book, *Essential Exercises for the Childbearing Years.*[1] In most other countries a formal medical approach to the rehabilitation of this condition is common.

Traditionally, physical therapists have been concerned with lesions of musculoskeletal tissues that have potential for disruption of function, movement, or alignment of the human form. Since diastasis recti fits the profile of a condition deserving a physical therapist's attention, its management should become the responsibility of the physical therapy profession.

Diastasis recti is defined as the separation of the rectus abdominis muscle (Fig. 3-1). The mechanics of this separation involve the widening of the linea alba. Historically, the obstetric community paid more attention to diastasis development and its management than does the present medical community. In the early 1900s, De Lee, Hirst, Crossen, Cooke, and Webster were a few of the medical authors who discussed the etiology and management of diastasis in their obstetric texts.[2-6] Rupture, enteroptosis, and visceroptosis were terms used synonymously at that time with diastasis recti.[2,3] These terms described a separation of the rectus muscle as a result of the linea alba giving way to the strain of an advancing pregnancy. Childbearing was always listed as the predisposing factor, especially when there was a succession of pregnancies. Corsets, for the nonpregnant as well as pregnant, were also credited as a primary factor in the development of a diastasis.[2,7,8] Presently, physicians who are concerned with the management of hernias also deal with diastasis recti. The simplest form of a ventral or epigastric hernia is in the region of the linea alba and represents a diastasis recti.[9,10] The significant difference between a true hernia and a diastasis is the presence of a hernial sac.[10] Specifically, with a diastasis recti, no break has occurred in the transversalis fascia that would

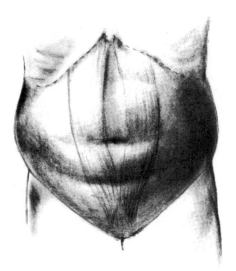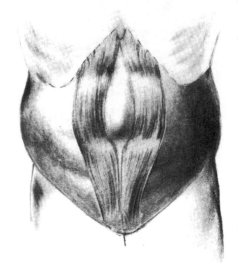

Fig. 3-1. Diagrammatic representations of diastasis recti.

allow the development of a sac with peritoneal contents. A diastasis recti can result in a bulge of the abdominal wall upon the increase of intra-abdominal pressure. However, the diastasis can just as often exist without this bulge. Iason defined three degrees of rectus separation: (1) Complete separation, in which the fibers of the linea alba are completely separated from the xiphoid cartilage to the symphysis pubis. Only skin and peritoneum are left as coverage over the abdominal viscera. (2) Incomplete/Complete separation, in which occurs a complete separation and division of the linea alba from the symphysis pubis to the umbilicus. The remaining fibers are normal or only partly separated above the umbilicus. (3) Incomplete separation, in which the fibers of the linea alba are attenuated or separated but not completely severed, leaving the linea alba greatly widened.[11]

Unfortunately, Iason did not document references to support these statements and no recent research has investigated the actual changes that constitute a separation.

The normal distance between the rectus bellies above the umbilicus is approximately 2 cm. Below the umbilicus the bellies are in contact with each other. Diastasis recti involves a separation of a distance greater than the normal anatomic separation at either level.

The plastic surgeon is another source of medical management of diastasis recti. Abdominoplasty is done to correct distended and pendulous abdominal skin and fat as well as to tighten relaxed and weakened abdominal muscles. Pregnancy, with its related abdominal changes, and post-obesity weight loss are the major indications for performing abdominoplasty.

This chapter discusses anatomy relevant to diastasis recti, the functional anatomy of the region, physiologic changes related to diastasis, its incidence, implications, and management. The authors hope that upon completing the chapter the reader will be more knowledgeable about diastasis and that the groundwork has been established to incorporate evaluation and treatment of diastasis recti into each individual therapist's practice.

ANATOMY

The anatomy most relevant to diastasis recti is that of the anterolateral abdominal wall, including the fascial layers, the four pairs of flat muscles, their aponeuroses, and the linea alba (Fig. 3-2). The linea alba is the result of the fusion of the right and left aponeuroses of the three pairs of anterolateral abdominal muscles in the midline from the sternum to the pubis. The fascial layers of the abdominal wall are divided into a superficial and deep layer. The superficial fascia, referred to as the fatty layer of Camper, is a single layer with varying amounts of fat. The deep fascial layer, also known as the membranous layer of Scarpa, is more membranous and contains elastic fibers. Aerolar tissue connects this layer to the aponeurosis of the external oblique muscle; medially, it is tightly adhered to the linea alba and symphysis pubis.

Aponeuroses are defined as flat sheets of densely arranged collagen fibers

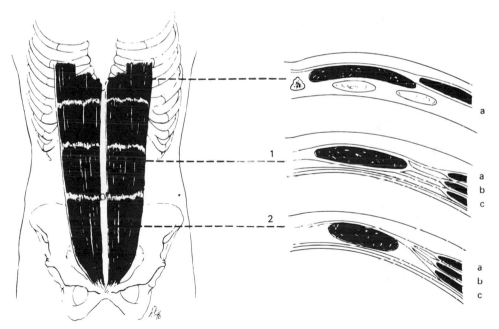

Fig. 3-2. Cross sections of rectus abdominus and its sheath. Above (1) and below (2) the arcuate line. External oblique (a), internal oblique (b), transversus abdominus (c). (Kendall F, McCreary E: Muscles Testing and Function. 3rd Ed. The Williams & Wilkins Co., Baltimore, 1983.)

usually consisting of several layers. Collagen fibers within each layer are parallel but can be aligned in different directions in adjacent layers. Interweaving of the fibrous bundles from one layer to another increases the aponeuroses' structural stability and perhaps their elasticity. Aponeuroses as regular connective tissue are primarily collagenous but may have a few elastic fibers around the collagen fibers. Essentially, aponeuroses are broad flat tendons.

The anterolateral muscle group of the abdomen consists of four pairs of large, flat, thin muscles. These muscles are the external and internal obliques, transversus abdominis, and rectus abdominis.

The external oblique is the largest and most superficial of the three muscles of the lateral abdominal wall. This broad, thin muscular sheet is composed of muscular tissue on the lateral wall and an aponeurosis on the anterior wall. It originates from the lower eight ribs and inserts on the iliac crest, the anterior iliac spine, the pubic tubercle, and by aponeurosis anteriorly into the linea alba. The fibers are directed downward and medially.

Internal to the external oblique is the internal oblique, which is also a broad, thin sheet of muscular tissue. This muscle arises from the thoracolumbar fascia, iliac crest, and inguinal ligament. The fibers extend upward and medially, coursing perpendicular to the fibers of the external oblique. Insertion of the internal oblique fibers is upon the cartilage of the seventh, eighth, and ninth ribs and also by aponeurosis into the linea alba.

The innermost and thinnest of the abdominal muscles is the transversus abdominis. As the name implies, the direction of its fibers is transverse; they pass directly forward and around the abdominal wall. This muscle arises from the inner surfaces of the lower six ribs, from the anterior internal aspect of the iliac crest, and from the inguinal ligament. The fibers terminate in an aponeurosis that inserts into the linea alba.

The linea alba is formed by decussating fibers of the aponeuroses of the three right and left flat lateral abdominal muscles and forms a tendinous raphe from the xiphoid process to the symphysis pubis. Below the umbilicus, the linea alba is a narrow line where the recti muscles come in contact with each other. Above the umbilicus, as a result of the diverging of the rectus bellies, the linea alba forms a band about 2 cm wide.

The rectus abdominis is the fourth muscle of the anterolateral abdominal wall. This long, straplike muscle extends the length of the anterior abdominal wall on each side of the linea alba. The rectus arises by two tendons from the pubic bone and its ligaments. The muscle belly widens as it extends upward to its insertion on the xiphoid process and the costal cartilages of the fifth, sixth, and seventh ribs.

The rectus abdominis is entirely enclosed in a sheath formed by the aponeuroses of the muscles of the lateral walls of the abdomen. At the lateral border of the rectus, above the umbilicus, the aponeurosis of the internal oblique divides into an anterior and a posterior layer. The anterior sheet blends with the aponeurosis of the external oblique and passes in front of the rectus. The posterior sheet passes behind the rectus and blends with the aponeurosis of the transversus. These layers unite at the medial border of the rectus to form the linea alba. Below the line of the umbilicus, the aponeuroses of all three flat muscles pass anterior to the rectus, leaving only the fascia of the transversus posterior to the rectus.

The anterior and posterior walls of the rectus sheath are extraordinary in that they are elastic in the vertical direction and inelastic in the transverse direction.[12] This specificity of function of the sheath is a result of the interlacement of the fibers of the aponeuroses that compose it. A major function of this feature is the rectus sheath's ability to adapt itself to the differences in the distance between the sternum and pubis during the various movements of the trunk. In addition to its adaptive capabilities, it provides a rigid inextensible tendon of insertion for the three anterolateral muscles that attach to it laterally. Imbedded in the anterior wall of the rectus sheath anterior to the rectus belly is the pyramidalis muscle, which originates anterior to the pubis and symphysis. This muscle extends upward, decreasing in size as it ascends, and terminates in a point on the linea alba midway between the umbilicus and pubis. This small, triangular, fleshy muscle is often absent. Its action is that of providing tension upon or reinforcment of the linea alba.[13] Its frequent absence may be implicated in diastasis seen below the umbilicus.

Functional Anatomy

The muscles of the abdominal wall along with the back extensors and gluteus maximus play a vital role in maintaining trunk stability.[14] The abdominals are also involved in relieving pressure on the lumbar intervertebral discs.[15,16] These functions of the abdominal muscles are in addition to the more traditional descriptions of their roles in trunk flexion, lateral flexion, trunk rotation, forced expiration, and pelvic girdle alignment.[17-23] The abdominals also collectively aid in increasing the intra-abdominal pressure necessary for defecation, urination, emessing, parturition, and expiration.[13,24] Taken together, this muscle group has important implications for daily activities such as rolling over, lifting, and elimination, as well as for maintenance of proper static posture. These implications of diastasis will be explored in another section of this chapter.

The abdominal muscles have some separate though often related functions which impact on the area of obstetrics and gynecology. Kendall and McCreary, when discussing the common action of the anterior fibers of the external obliques, the lower anterior fibers of the internal obliques, and the transversus, cite their role in compression and support of the abdominal viscera.[22] The transversus also plays a role in stabilizing the linea alba due to its course and attachments.[22] Weakness of the rectus abdominis or obliqui permits an anterior pelvic tilt with resulting lordotic posture. The effect of transversus abdominis weakness on posture is less direct but present all the same; it permits a bulging of the anterior abdominal wall and tends to affect an increase in lordosis.[22] During straining or bearing down against a closed glottis, the obliques appear to respond by protecting the inguinal region, supposedly against herniation.[17]

Lastly, the rectus sheath is thought to protect the abdominal area occupied by the rectus abdominis during activities which increase intra-abdominal pressure, including, of course, second stage pushing.[17,23] A void exists in the literature relative to either electromyographic or manual testing of muscle function of the abdomen during pregnancy. Even less information can be found regarding the adominals of those pregnant women who present with a diastasis.

PHYSIOLOGIC CHANGES RELATED TO DIASTASIS

Numerous physiologic changes occur during the childbearing year that impact upon the incidence and etiology of diastasis recti. Those to be briefly explored in this chapter are the hormonal alterations and their impact on connective tissue, the increasing mechanical stress placed upon the abdominal wall and upon the linea alba, and the changing functional capacities of the abdominal muscles with advancing pregnancy and in the postpartum period.

Among the alterations in hormonal levels during the childbearing year are increased levels of estrogen, progesterone, and relaxin. Aside from their effect upon the reproductive tract, these hormones are commonly implicated in the softening of connective tissue that is believed to occur throughout the body during this period.[1,25,26] Moore states that connective tissue becomes less supportive as a result of increasing levels of estrogen, progesterone, and relaxin during pregnancy.[26] She attributes this to a loosening of the abdominal fascia and to reduced cohesion between collagen fibers.

Maternal Hormones

In the past few years relaxin has received a great deal of attention and many have attempted to credit this peptide hormone with all the generalized relaxation of soft tissues that begins in pregnancy and remains throughout the postpartum period. Recent research on humans has substantiated relaxin's role in the softening of tissues only in the reproductive tract (cervix and uterus). MacLennan, in an extensive review on the role of relaxin in human reproduction, stresses the fact that relaxin affects only those tissues which possess target sites specific to this hormone. To date, these have been found only in the cervix, myometrium, decidua, and breast connective tissue. The facilitation of remodeling of the connective tissue in these structures is thought to allow the necessary changes for pregnancy and parturition. Animal studies do suggest relaxin to be responsible for connective tissue changes in other tissues, specially throughout the pelvic girdle, but these studies cannot yet be extrapolated to humans. Relaxin appears to influence collagen metabolism in most target tissues. It stimulates collagen biosynthesis and decreases the viscosity of the ground substance, thereby increasing the extensibility and remodelling of the tissue. Evidence also indicates that a relationship exists between estrogen and relaxin in regards to hormonal priming. The estrogen/progesterone ratio may mediate relaxin's effects. MacLennan does not suggest any direct effect of relaxin on structures such as the linea alba but admits that the research accomplished so far is in its infancy.[27]

Interesting to note is that relaxin has recently been shown to appear in the pregnant woman 14 days after conception, is highest during the first trimester, decreases by 20 percent after that period, and remains steady throughout the rest of pregnancy. Unlike animals, no preparturition surge is found. Levels return to prepregnancy norm by day 3 postpartum irregardless of the woman's lactational status.[28,29] In the literature, controversy exists as to whether or not relaxin is produced in the nonpregnant woman during the menstrual cycle. One consensus is that if relaxin is produced, it is at much lower levels than in the pregnant state.[29,30]

The proportions of progesterone and estrogen during pregnancy are diametrically opposed to those of relaxin; unlike relaxin, they rise as pregnancy progresses. These hormones are initially secreted by the corpus luteum. As levels of chorionic gonadatropin (the hormone responsible for continued maintenance of the corpus luteum) diminish, placental output of estrogen and progesterone increase. This leads to a marked increase of blood steroid levels during the last 6 months of pregnancy.

At present, although the exact hormones responsible for soft tissue laxity observed during the childbearing year remains unclear, the normal groundwork has been clarified and possible mechanisms have been proposed. The histologic impact of these hormonal changes upon the linea alba has not been researched, but grounded theory supports the belief that hormonal changes and increasing mechanical stress upon the abdominal wall combine to allow diastasis to occur.

Mechanical Stress During Pregnancy

The mechanical stresses placed upon the structures of the abdominal wall, including the linea alba and the muscle themselves, result from the increasing size of the fetus and its necessary support system. The uterus itself increases in size from 6.5 cm long, 4 cm wide and 2.5 cm deep to 32 cm long, 24 cm wide and 22 cm deep. The weight of the uterus increases from 50 g before pregnancy to 1000 g at term. When at term, the uterus contains the fetus, placenta, and more than 1,000 ml of amniotic fluid (compared to a prepregnancy capacity of only 2 cc), amounting to a weight of approximately 12 lbs.[31] A method of monitoring these changes externally is found in Bartholomew's "rule of fourths," which establishes a correlation between fundal height and duration of pregnancy.[26] The fundus of the uterus is reported to be at the height of the pubis at the end of the first month, at the level of the umbilicus at the end of the fifth month (20 weeks), and then one-fourth of the distance to the xiphoid process at the end of each of the following months. A slight drop in the height of the fundus may be noted in the ninth month secondary to "lightening," or a slight descent of the fetus into the bony pelvis. Significant to note is that a recent study on the incidence of diastasis recti demonstrated a relationship between advancing pregnancy and the development of diastasis.[32] The diastasis is not theorized to be solely due to the increasing mechanical stress of the uterus upon the abdominal wall, but this stress factor (probably coupled with the hormonal changes already discussed) is believed to play an important role in the etiology of this condition.

The growth of the fetus has an indirect effect upon the abdominal wall as well. Much displacement of the abdominal organs occurs during the later part of pregnancy, which thereby adds to the amount of stress placed upon the abdominal wall. Additionally, significant alteration in the ribcage dimensions places tension upon the abdominal muscles, which have their attachments on the ribs. The anterior-posterior and transverse diameters of the chest are increased by 2 cm.[31,33]

During pregnancy the fetus, its supporting environment, and the abdominal organs place prolonged stress upon the linea alba. Frankel and Nordin discussed the concept of "creep" as it relates to connective tissue.[34] When soft tissues are subjected to "constant low loading over an extended period of time, slow deformation of the soft tissues, or creep takes place."[34] Laban discusses similar findings; he terms the initial response to stress "elastic-like," and states that maintained stress yields a period of "plastic-like" deformation.[35] Entrance into the plastic phase implies a permanent change, or at least a long recovery time after removal of the deforming stress. With these alterations, on a molecular level one would see a structural change resulting in the breaking of bonds.[36] Molecular changes in the elastic phase would result in a change in alignment; that is, the collagen fibers would become straighter and more longitudinally oriented.[36] The nine months of pregnancy certainly produce a prolonged, sustained stress, thus subjecting the linea alba to the manifestations of the creep phenomenon. Still unclear is whether this prolonged stress results in a permanent elongation of the connective tissue of the linea alba or adjacent fascia or whether actual loss of integrity or severance of the tissues occurs.

Abdominal Muscle Function

Finally, among the physiologic changes that relate to diastasis recti are changes in the function of abdominal muscles. There is a lack of research quantifying the differences in electromyogram (EMG) output between the abdominal musculature of the nonpregnant woman and that of the pregnant woman. No research reports measurements of the EMG output of the abdominal muscles of a woman who exhibits a diastasis. Some research, however, suggests that the function of abdominal musculature in the pregnant woman is different from that of the nonpregnant woman. In 1980, Booth studied nonpregnant women at 38 weeks gestation and women at 6 weeks postpartum (30 per group) to determine which of some commonly performed abdominal exercises would be most efficient in terms of EMG output.[37] Of interest here was the finding that, in pregnancy, a markedly greater number of effective exercises for the abdominals were noted than the number that were deemed effective for the nonpregnant population. By 5 days postpartum the data began to return to nonpregnant levels. By 6 weeks postpartum the change was complete.

The article does not speculate as to why the abdominals of pregnant women are recruited in movements in which they do not usually participate, but it is clear that their function is somewhat altered during pregnancy. Unclear at this time is the question of how altered mechanics or strength of the abdominals may affect the development of diastasis, but Booth's study does offer the obstetric/gynecologic (OB/GYN) physical therapist additional abdominal strengthening exercises from which to select when caring for a woman who exhibits a diastasis prenatally or shortly after delivery.[37]

In 1978, Spence manually tested muscle strength of 40 postpartum women.[38] She found that pregnancy reduced the strength of the abdominals, though not significantly, and that a trend toward greater weakness was noted in multiparas versus primiparas. Spence measured strength in only three women with a diastasis greater than 2 cm; but of those, she found one to exhibit 80 percent normal strength of the rectus and two to present with 60 percent normal strength of the rectus.[38]

Clinically, of course, in the third trimester and immediately postpartum, many pregnant women subjectively present with weakened abdominals. Again, how this weakness contributes to development of diastasis and to prevention requires further study.

ETIOLOGY

The inner surfaces of the abdominal recti, from the umbilicus down to the pubes, lie flush to each other, nothing separating them except their sheathes in the male sex and in non-child-bearing women. On the contrary, however, with the mothers of one or more children, there may be a well-marked interval dividing these muscles, varying from one to several inches. Pregnancy, in many women of modern life, over-fed and under-exercised, whose foetuses are large, fat and plump, puts the muscular plane of the abdomen on a great strain, often so much over-stretching them that they never quite recover their tonicity after labor, or the fibrous structures are so far over-stretched that a complete return to their former integrity is quite impossible. The mother then is left "pot-bellied." The belly hangs over the pubic brim. The recti muscles have so far diverged, as to permit the greater part of the abdominal contents to occupy this hiatus, caused by the want of muscular support. With women so burdened, if there be but little adipose tissue present, we may at times quite distinctly feel the vermicular movements of the intestine through the thinned integument. These bulging masses in the lower mesial plane, like those above, are not attended with any danger to life. They are not commonly classified as herniae, though aetiologically and pathologically they are identical. They derive their greatest interest from the deforming effects which they produce, and from the fact that many of the most aggravated cases of this description, if seen in young women, may be averted or wholly cured by simple means.

The preceding is an excerpt from Thomas Manley's *Hernia: Its Palliative and Radical Treatment in Adults, Children and Infants,* published in 1893.[39] Interesting to note is the extensive insight Manley had into the etiology of diastasis. Common to discussions regarding the causes of diastasis, both in the past and at this time, is consideration of parity. (By parity we mean pregnancy carried to a point of viability, regardless of outcome.) Accounts regarding pregnancy as a cause of diastasis report that the recti separate as a result of the distension of the abdomen. Manley more specifically discusses the "over-stretching" of the muscular planes of the abdomen.[39] A current explanation is provided by Kendall's discussion of stretch weakness.[22] Stretch weakness is the result of muscles being maintained in an elongated position beyond their neutral physiologic rest position for a prolonged period of time. (Mechanical stresses related to the development of diastasis are discussed in more detail in the section on physiologic changes related to pregnancy.) Manley even alludes to the "creep" phenomenon (also discussed previously) when he refers to the fibrous structures being so far "over-stretched" that they are unable to return to their former state.[39] Several theories discussed in this chapter describe the role hormones play in increasing the laxity of fibrous tissues.

Any condition that results in a persistent excessive increase in intra-abdominal pressure favors the development of a diastasis.[24] The presence of the gravid uterus within the abdominal cavity automatically increases the intra-abdominal pressure.[2] Situations during pregnancy that increase the pressure above this level would most certainly predispose the woman to the development of a diastasis. Such situations would include lifting or carrying heavy objects. A sudden strain or fall may also be the starting point of a diastasis. A decrease in the tone of the tissues of the abdominal wall as a result of general weakness or emaciation may also predispose one to diastasis development.

Even though many factors can be associated with the development of diastasis, pregnancy is the most important.

INCIDENCE

While diastasis recti is not a condition limited to pregnant or postpartum women, it is most often discussed in that context. Diastasis can also be seen in obese, hypersthenic males, in patients with chronic lung disease, and in children.

In children the linea alba is thinner and wider than in the adult. Diastasis here appears as an ovoid or elongated midepigastric swelling which manifests upon exertion. As the child ages and his abdominal muscles increase in size and strength, the diastasis decreases in magnitude until the two sides of the rectus reach their adult orientation.

By far the greatest incidence of diastasis recti is found among the population of women during the childbearing year. Boissonnault, in a recent study entitled, "The Incidence of Diastasis Recti During the Childbearing Year," investigated incidence across six groups of women of childbearing age.[32] The first group of women tested were those of childbearing age (18–35) who had never been pregnant. The second, third, and fourth groups consisted of pregnant women in their first, second, and third trimesters, respectively. The fifth and sixth groups were composed of postpartum women. Group five consisted of those women who were immediately postpartum (up to 72 hours postpartum), and the sixth group consisted of women who were between 5 weeks and 3 months postpartum. Only women who had had no back or abdominal surgery, had no history of connective tissue disease, did not participate in regular abdominal exercise, had singleton vertex presentations (appropriate to third trimester and postpartum subjects), and term vaginal deliveries (if postpartum) were included as subjects.

In testing, each subject was asked to raise her head and shoulders off of the table until the spines of the scapulae left the table, as palpated by the researcher's hand) (Fig. 3-3).

Once in this position, the author measured for diastasis by placing her fingers horizontally across the linea alba and determining how many fingers fit into the space between the borders of the two recti bellies (Fig. 3-4).

Measurements were taken above, below, and at the umbilicus. Diastasis was classified as present or absent according to Noble's criteria; a measurement of two fingers or less was considered normal, and a measurement greater than two fingers was considered to indicate a diastasis.[1] This measurement technique has proven unreliable when employed by different raters, but since one researcher conducted all measurements, unreliability was not a factor.[40]

Statistical analysis of the data on the 89 women in this study revealed a significant relationship between a woman's membership in one of the six groups and the presence of diastasis. A women's placement in the course of pregnancy had an effect on whether or not she was likely to develop a diastasis. No diastasis was found in groups 1 and 2 (the nonpregnant and first trimester subjects). The presence of diastasis first appeared in group 3 (the second trimester women), and peaked in group 4 (the third trimester subjects). The presence of diastasis remained high in the immediate postpartum group and declined with group 6 (the latter postpartum group), though levels did not return to the base line of zero seen in groups 1 and 2. Twenty-seven percent of the second trimester women tested presented with diastasis, while 66 percent of the third trimester women, 53 percent of the immediate postpartum women, and 36 percent of the later postpartum group demonstrated diastasis. Bursch reported that 62.5 percent of the postpartum women she tested (up to 92 hours post delivery) demonstrated diastasis of greater than two finger widths.[40] Spence found 50 percent of 6 week postpartum women she tested had diastasis, but the classification criteria were unclear.[38]

Some disagreement exists as to the location of diastasis along the linea alba. Ponka reports that the separation is most common below the umbilicus in multiparous women, while Noble believes it is most common at the umbilicus.[1,24] In the majority of cases Boissonnault found the separation to be at the

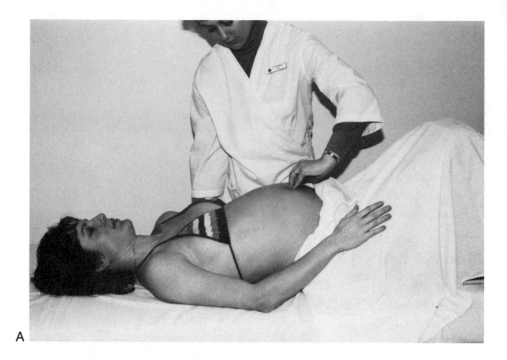

A

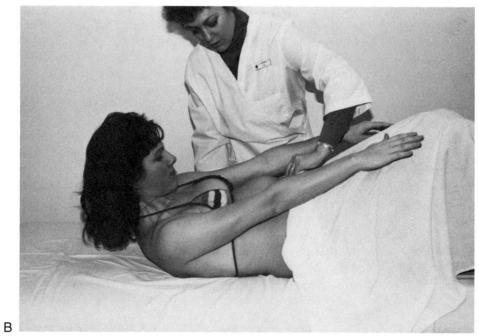

B

Fig. 3-3.   Testing for diastasis recti. **(A)** Starting position. **(B)** Final position.

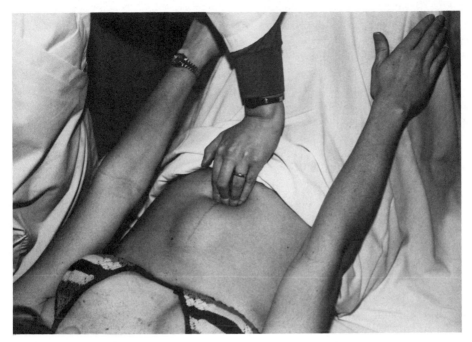

Fig. 3-4. The patient shown has a four finger diastasis recti.

umbilicus, although she sometimes found it alone and sometimes saw it in conjunction with separation above the umbilicus as well.[32] Additionally, separation above the umbilicus did occur quite often by itself. Only four subjects out of those who demonstrated a diastasis had one below the umbilicus, and all of these were seen in conjunction with separation in one of the other two regions as well.

In terms of clinical relevance, the authors state with some certainty that the incidence of diastasis recti remains high enough in the postpartum population to warrant medical intervention. This problem does not necessarily resolve itself spontaneously, and the condition should not be thought normal. Rather, it should be treated as a pathologic condition. Additionally, although the separation is most common at the umbilicus, therapists should palpate along the entire linea alba when screening for its presence.

THE IMPLICATIONS OF DIASTASIS RECTI

The implications of a diastasis recti left unresolved fall into two categories; one relates to cosmesis of the abdomen and the other to abdominal weakness and its effect on function, posture, and low back pain.

Cosmetically, diastasis is rarely a problem by itself. Only when diastasis presents as a component in a larger syndrome involving a pendulous, weakened abdomen with lax, striated skin is cosmesis an issue.[12,41,42] One author has noted diastasis recti as the primary cause in this syndrome in 3 out of 300 cases studied, or only 1 percent.[42] In *Plastic Surgery of the Abdomen* Elbaz noted diastasis to be a common component of the many significant changes that can occur in a woman's physique: ". . . pregnancy frequently causes wrinkled, strained and distended abdomens with many stretch marks. . . . The skin around the umbilicus appears 'waffled,' the abdominal wall is relaxed, and a major diastasis of the rectus muscles occurs."[12] The treatment for the larger cosmetic problem will be discussed later. Functionally, a diastasis of any significance (according to Noble, greater than 2 finger widths; according to Elbaz, greater than 4 cm) will likely impair both the strength and effectiveness of the rectus abdominis and perhaps do the same to the other muscles of the abdominal wall as well, since their aponeuroses decussate at the linea alba.[1,12] Any change in orientation of the linea alba should effect the ability of these muscles to manifest their normal mechanics. Fascial structures in and around the abdominal muscles like the linea alba and the rectus sheath assist in the coherence of the contracting parts. The loss of this assistance results in the loss of the cumulative strength of the individual muscles, and as a result muscular energy is dissipated.[11] This decreased efficiency may result in dysfunction and disability from loss of the muscles as force attenuates, from abnormal posture, and from activities of daily living (ADL) impairment.

As was mentioned earlier, the abdominal muscles are important in lending support to the rest of the trunk and to the pelvic viscera. A relationship exists between contraction of the abdominal musculature and the amount of force placed upon the structures of the spine, especially when lifting.[15,16] Lifting an object forces an immediate valsalva maneuver which stabilizes the thoraco-abdominal cavity by contraction of the expiratory muscles, including the abdominals. The rise in pressure transforms the cavity into a rigid cylinder lying anterior to the vertebral column. This aids in reducing the axial compression forces acting on the intervertebral discs by transferring these forces to the bony pelvis and perineum. Thus, weakness or inefficiency of the abdominal muscles may be implicated in spinal dysfunction, since the discs of the lumber spine may have to accommodate more force than they are able to withstand.

Abnormal posture—specifically, abnormal alignment of the pelvis on the lower extremities or of the trunk on the pelvis—potentially contributes to development of low back pain and/or dysfunction.[23,15] The anterior pelvic tilt resulting from rectus abdominis weakness and the bulging of the anterior abdominal wall due to transversus weakness both increase lumbar lordosis. The resulting altered mechanics of the trunk may lead to soft tissue imbalances and/or joint disturbances.

Among the more direct results of abdominal muscle impairment are those that relate to the patient's ability to perform activities of daily living. The primary actions of the abdominal muscles are those of trunk flexion, rotation, and lateral bending. Inability to fully accomplish these tasks surely restricts a patient's independence. Bed mobility, dressing, and transfers all require normal abdominal strength in order to be performed without assistance or adaptation. Interestingly, large and probably longstanding diastases have been found in elderly women each of whose independent ADL status has been compromised. Further research is needed to clarify the role of diastasis in impairment of these functions.

No less important in terms of quality of life is the function of the abdominals in activities which require increases in intra-abdominal pressure, specifically, voiding, defecating, emessing, and the delivering of a fetus. When the thorax and pelvis are fixed, the abdominal muscles, especially the obliqui, exert compressive force on the abdominal viscera. This force aids in the accomplishment of those activities listed above.[13,24] Inefficiency of these muscles, then, may interfere with this mechanism.

Protection of abdominal and pelvic viscera is another function of the abdominal wall. Some of this wall's ability to splint this region could be lost in the presence of diastasis. More directly, a severe diastatis leaves the abdominal contents (including a fetus) quite vulnerable, as all that may be between them and the outside world is peritonium and skin.[12]

Presently, discussion of these potentially grave implications of diastasis are purely speculative. The role of the abdominal musculature in these areas has been well researched, but the effect of diastasis on the efficiency and strength of these muscles has not. Logically, however, based on anatomic relationships, one may assume that impairment of the linea alba will be detrimental to the normal function of the abdominal muscles and potentiate dysfunction, as discussed above.

MANAGEMENT OF DIASTASIS RECTI

Management of diastasis recti ranges from the conservative approach of external support and exercise to the extreme of surgical repair.

Early references state that prevention of diastasis is the best cure. De Lee, in his 1920 text *Obstetrics for Nurses,* states, "To prevent muscular insufficiency, one must begin with the girl. She should develop herself as does the boy, with active sports, rowing, swimming, climbing, etc. Health exercise of the whole body should form part of her daily routine."[43] As far back as 1893, Manley made a specific reference to pregnant women being "under exercised" and cited this as a precipitating factor in the development of diastasis recti.[39] This finding lends significant support to prenatal exercises for prevention of diastasis, but as therapists, we also deal with the condition as its exists.

The most common treatment discussed by the early authors was the incorporation of an external support (an abdominal binder or corset) and exercise. Several functions of the abdominal binder were indicated. One was to transmit the superincumbent weight from the muscles and aponeuroses to the vertebral column.[39] Cooke lists three functions of the abdominal binder: (1) prevention of hemorrhage; (2) prevention of cerebral anaemia; and (3) prevention of diastasis by approximating the recti muscles of the abdomen.

Associated with the use of the abdominal binder was an exercise program to strengthen the abdominals.[1-3,39,43] Noble describes a specific exercise for decreasing or arresting the separation of the recti bellies and increasing the tone of the abdominals without increasing intra-abdominal pressure. This involves the patient assuming a hook lying position. The patient's hands are across the abdomen pulling the muscles to the midline as the patient raises her head. Emphasis is given to slow exhalation during the activity to prevent an increase in intra-abdominal pressure. Breath holding would cause the intra-abdominal pressure to increase and facilitate the bulging of a diastasis.

When the diastasis is reduced with the above correction technique exercise, progression is determined by the level of abdominal strength. The exercise can be made more difficult by altering the position of the arms, legs, and trunk.[1,22]

In a study by Fransman–van Santen, Noble's method of diastasis correction was found to be effective when done in combination with a posterior pelvic tilt.[1,44] Fransman–van Santen found that EMG activity was greater in the rectus abdominis when head lifting was done in conjunction with a posterior pelvic tilt.[44] The diastasis corrective exercise with a posterior tilt was done by 20 women 10 times a day on the second through the sixth day postpartum. The only other instructions given were to maintain a posterior tilt as much as possible. Compared to 20 women who also had diastasis but did not exercise, a marked reduction in the diastasis magnitude was found in the posterior pelvic tilt group.

According to Ponka, prior to correction of a diastasis, maximum improvement in pulmonary function is necessary so that excessive intra-abdominal pressure is avoided. This finding relates to the tendency of patients to hold their breath on exertion during exercise and other activities. Instruction should be given to patients to exhale during exercise to prevent excessive increased intra-abdominal pressure from holding the breath.

In the etiology section of this chapter stretch weakness is discussed as a causative factor in the development of diastasis recti. Stretch weakness is the effect on muscles which comes from their remaining in an elongated position beyond the neutral physiologic rest position.[22] Essential to the treatment is realignment of the parts to achieve a neutral position. Noble is attempting to achieve this realignment by having patients place their hands across the abdomen and pull the muscles toward the midline.[1] This technique is appropriate in theory, but unfortunately has not been substantiated with research. Kendall states that the use of supportive measures to reestablish and maintain normal alignment until the weakened muscles are rehabilitated is an important factor in the treatment of stretch weakness.[22] The therapist might at least consider some means of support in the early rehabilitative stages of diastasis recti.

Historically, electrotherapy has been a significant component in the conservative management of diastasis. Techniques have varied greatly. In the late 1800s, electrification of the abdominal wall with injections of strychnine into the muscles, massage, and "douching sedulously" comprised a popular treatment regime to reestablish tonicity of the abdominal wall.[39] Fortunately this treatment protocol has not withstood the test of time.

As time passed, electrotherapy management progressed to a state more familiar to today's physical therapists. Massey's *Conservative Gynecology and Electro-Therapeutics* appeared in 1905. In it Massey describes a treatment regime similar to procedures used today. Electric current of sufficient strength to induce contraction was applied to the weakened muscles. The current had to be from 100 to 150 mA. It was combined with a powerful primary induction (faradic) current applied from an active pad on the abdomen to a large dispersive pad beneath the patient. This approach provides a basis for the present physical therapist to utilize electrical stimulation as part of a treatment program for a diastasis recti. Further research must yet be done to support the use of electrical modalities in facilitating and reeducating the abdominal wall with a diastasis.

Surgical management of diastasis recti is most often done in connection with a hernia repair or abdominoplasty. Abdominal plastic surgery is becoming more popular with today's population. Abdominoplasty is surgery used to correct deformations of the abdomen. This surgical technique involves removal of distended and pendulous skin and fat. If a diastasis is present, it is repaired by suturing the rectus bellies together. Management following surgical repair includes wearing an abdominal support for one month postoperatively. Abdominal strengthening exercises are initiated at the end of the first month after surgery.

As discussed previously, conservative management in the past focused on external support, exercise, and electrotherapy. All of these methods of management are within the realm of physical therapy. Our responsibility is to do the research that supports utilization of specific treatment techniques in the management of diastasis recti. As the role of physical therapy in diastasis management is established, it is hoped that the profession will be instrumental in decreasing the need for more radical approaches.

CONCLUSIONS

Diastasis recti, or the separation of the rectus abdominis muscle at the linea alba, is a condition which warrants the attention of the physical therapist working with the obstetric population. The etiology of this condition remains unproven, but grounded theory suggests a causative relationship between the mechanical stresses placed upon the abdominal wall due to the increasing size of the fetus, the resultant stretch weakness of the abdominal musculature, and the alteration of connective tissue due to maternal hormones. Diastasis is uncommon in women of childbearing age who have not been pregnant. The condition first appears in the obstetric population during the second trimester of pregnancy and is found most frequently in women in their third trimester. Postpartum incidence remains high initially and declines in the latter postpartum period, though not to prepregnancy norms. Diastasis is most commonly noted at the umbilicus but can be seen anywhere along the length of the linea alba.

The functional consequences of an unresolved diastasis remain theoretical. If separation of the recti bellies impairs the function of the abdominals, then the implications for dysfunction are wide-ranging. Problems include difficulties with activities requiring increases in intra-abdominal pressure (parturition, elimination, etc.), trunk flexion, rotation, side bending, loss of support to the abdominal viscera, as well as the potential to develop back pain due to faulty posture or abnormal trunk mechanics.

Prevention and rehabilitation of diastasis recti falls directly under the auspices of the physical therapist. As diastasis is a condition affecting the musculoskeletal tissue with repercussions to the musculoskeletal system, physical therapists must take responsibility to see that effective preventive and rehabilitative treatment programs are researched and instituted. Currently, prenatal noninvasive treatment focuses on preventing an already present diastasis from worsening while maintaining as much strength as possible in the abdominal musculature. Postpartum treatment involves strengthening the rectus abdominis in order to reapproximate the two bellies without increasing intra-abdominal pressure. Current prevention focuses on preparing a woman's abdominal musculature through performance of accepted abdominal strengthening exercises for the physiologic and anatomic changes it will undergo during pregnancy.[32]

Much of what has been written in this chapter has been speculative. What is clear is that diastasis recti is present in sufficient number beyond the initial postpartum period to warrant further research. Future research must focus on etiology and prevention of the problem as well as on the most efficient means of rehabilitating the separated recti muscles after delivery. Additionally, the implications of a diastasis recti should be explored through the use of electromyography of the abdominal musculature in subjects with this separation.

Hopefully, future investigation into the area of diastasis recti will provide the physical therapist with the necessary tools to develop a comprehensive approach to the care of the abdominal wall of women during and before they enter the childbearing year.

ACKNOWLEDGMENTS

We would like to thank William Boissonnault, M.S., P.T., and Lorraine Gohr, M.S., P.T., for their assistance with the photography and Teena J. Caliendo for the artwork.

REFERENCES

1. Noble E: Essential Exercises for the Childbearing Year. Houghton-Mifflin, Boston, 1982
2. DeLee J: The Principle and Practice of Obstetrics. 6th Ed. WB Saunders, 1933
3. Hirst J: A Manual of Gynecology. WB Saunders, Philadelphia, 1925

4. Crossen H: Diseases of Women. 6th Ed. CV Mosby, St. Louis, 1926
5. Cooke J: A Nurses Handbook of Obstetrics. 10th Ed. JB Lippincott, Philadelphia, 1924
6. Webster J: Textbook of Diseases of Women. WB Saunders, Philadelphia, 1907
7. Massey G: Conservative Gynecology and Electro-Therapeutics. FA Davis, Philadelphia, 1905
8. Anspach B: Gynecology. JB Lippincott, Philadelphia, 1921
9. Culbertson C: Surgery of the females pelvis. Gynecological and Obstetrical Monographs 15:211, 1931
10. Zimmerman L: Anatomy and Surgery of Hernia. Williams & Wilkins, Baltimore, 1953
11. Iason A: Sypnosis of Hernia. Grune & Stratton, New York, 1949
12. Elbaz J, Flageul G: Plastic Surgery of the Abdomen. Masson, New York, 1979
13. Williams P, Warwick R (eds.): 36th British Ed. WB Saunders, New York, 1980
14. Porterfield J: Dynamic stabilization of the trunk. Journal of Orthopedic and Sports Physical Therapy 6:271, 1985
15. Bartelink J: The role of abdominal pressure in relieving the pressure on the lumbar vertebral disc. J Bone Joint Surg 39:718, 1957
16. Kapandji I: The Physiology of Joints. Vol. 3. The Trunk and Vertebral Column. Churchill Livingstone, Edinburgh, 1974
17. Flloyd W, Silver P: Electromyopgrahic study of patterns of activity of the anterior abdominal wall muscles in man. J Anat 84:132–145, 1950
18. Flint M, Gudgell J: Electromyographic study of abdominal muscular activity during exercise. Research Quarterly 36:29, 1965
19. Gofrey K, Kondig L, Windell E: Electromyographic study of duration of muscle activity in sit-up variations. Arch Phys Med Rehabil 58:132, 1965
20. Partridge M, Walters C: Participation of the abdominal muscles in various moments of the trunk in man. Physical Therapy Review 39:791, 1959
21. Sheffield F, Major M: Electromyographic study of the abdominal muscles in in walking and other movements. Am J Phys Med 41:142, 1962
22. Kendall F, McCreary E: Muscles Testing and Function. 3rd Ed. Williams & Wilkins, Baltimore, 1983
23. Basmajian J: Muscles Alive. 3rd Ed. Williams & Wilkins, Baltimore, 1974
24. Ponka J: Hernias of the Abdominal Wall. WB Saunders, Philadelphia, 1980
25. Artal R, Wiswell: Exercise in Pregnancy. Williams & Wilkins, Baltimore, 1986
26. Moore M: Realties in Childbearing. WB Saunders, Philadelphia, 1983
27. MacLennan A: The role of relaxin in human reproduction. Clin Reprod Fertil 2:77, 1983
28. Weiss G: Relaxin. Annu Rev Physiol 46:42, 1984
29. O'Byrne E, Carriere B, Sorensen L, et al: Plasma immunoreactive relaxin levels in pregnant and non-pregnant women. J Clin Endocrinol Metab 47:1106, 1978
30. Loumaye E, Depreester S, Donnez J et al: Immunoreactive relaxin surge in the peritoneal fluid of women during the mid-luteal phase. Fertil Steril 42:856, 1984
31. Reeder S, Mastrainni L, Martin L et al: Maternity Nursing. 15th Ed. JB Lippincott, Philadelphia, 1980
32. Boissonnault J: The incidence of diastasis during the childbearing year. Unpublished manuscript, 1986
33. Lerch C, Bliss V: Maternity Nursing. 3rd Ed. CV Mosby, St. Louis, 1978
34. Frankel V, Nordin M: Basis Biomechanics of the Skeletal System. Lea & Febiger, Philadelphia, 1980

35. Laban M: Collagen tissue: implications of tis response to stress in vitro. Arch Phys Med Rehabil 43:461, 1962
36. Fung Y: Biomechanics, Mechanical Properties of Living Tissues. Springer-Verlag, New York, 1981
37. Booth D, Chennelle M, Jones D et al: Assessment of abdominal muscle exercises in non-pregnant, pregnant and post-partum subjects using electromyography. Australian Journal of Physiology 26.5:177, 1980
38. Spence M: Post Natal Survey. Australian Journal of Physiology 24:151, 1978
39. Manley T: Hernia: Its Pallative and Radical Treatment in Adults, Children and Infants. The Medical Press, Philadelphia, 1893
40. Bursch S: Interrater reliability of diastasis recti abdominis measurement. Phys Ther 67:1077, 1987
41. Fischel R: Vertical abdominoplasty. Plast Reconstr Surg 51:139, 1973
42. Pitanguy V: Abdominal lipectomy: an approach to it through an analysis of 300 consecutive cases. Plast Reconstr Surg 40:384,
43. DeLee J: Obstetrics for Nurses. 5th Ed. WB Saunders, Philadelphia, 1929
44. Fransman-van Santen T: Strengthening of the abdominal muscles for the patient with a diastasis recti. Nederlands Tijsdhrift voor Fysiotherapie 94:93–95

4 | Urogenital Dysfunction

Hollis Herman

Evaluation and treatment of the patient with urogenital dysfunction challenges the physical therapist to apply knowledge of anatomy, neurophysiology, pathology, and kinesiology to urologic, gynecologic, obstetric, and orthopedic conditions. While urogenital dysfunction is characteristically not emphasized in most physical therapy school curriculums, only physical therapists possess the necessary combined knowledge and skills in kinesiology, electrotherapy, and exercise science to address and treat problems in this area.[1,2]

Physical therapists currently working in obstetrics and gynecology should be aware of the role of the pelvic floor musculature in urogenital dysfunction. The majority of problems of urogenital dysfunction occur during childbearing or the childbearing years.

During labor and delivery, drastic changes occur in the anatomic position and shape of the pelvic muscles, viscera, and perineum. Stretching, tearing, and attenuation of the fascia and muscles occur. The pudendal and pelvic nerves may become partially denervated by traction or entrapment, resulting in laxity of the perineal muscles and sphincters.[3,4] Laxity of the musculature of the pelvic diaphragm in women (specifically the levator ani muscles) is the cause of prolapse of the pelvic organs,[5,6] decreased or absent sexual satisfaction,[7-9] and urinary incontinence.[10-13] Estimates range from 20 to 50 percent that all women suffer from some degree of incontinence of either congenital or traumatic origin.[7,14]

Urogenital dysfunction may arise from conditions and events that contribute to pelvic floor laxity or excessive tension. Excessive tension in the pelvic floor musculature has been cited as a possible factor in vaginismus,[15,16] dyspareunia,[16,17] pelvic pain and pressure, and urinary tract infections.[15]

This chapter focuses on urogenital dysfunctions most commonly found in women during the childbearing years. However, it is important for the reader to realize that neurologic, geriatric, and orthopedic clients can be affected as well. Urogenital dysfunctions are socially embarrassing, physically debilitating, and sexually inhibiting. The lifestyles of the clients as well as their families can be

83

profoundly affected by these dysfunctions. As musculoskeletal experts, physical therapists are an integral part of the health care team needed to assess and treat these dysfunctions.

ANATOMY

Discrepancies regarding the anatomy of the pelvic cavity are common. Therefore, a review of the anatomy and clarification of terms seems essential.

In many texts, the phrase "pelvic floor muscles" refers singularly to the levator ani muscles. However, according to Kegel[4] the pelvic floor consists of five layers of muscles and fascia attached to the bony ring of the pelvis. From superficial to deep the layers are as follows:

1. Superficial outlet muscles (anal sphincter only)
2. Urogenital triangle (urogenital diaphragm, vaginal and urethral sphincters)
3. Pelvic diaphragm (levator ani muscles)
4. Smooth muscle diaphragm
5. Endopelvic diaphragm

Urogenital Triangle

The urogenital triangle stretches from the ischial spines to the anterior wall of the pelvis and contains the external genitalia of the female, four layers of fascia, and two layers of muscle.[18] The superficial transverse perineal, the bulbocavernosus, and the ischiocavernosus muscles lie in the superficial layer.

The superficial transverse perineal muscle inserts into the perineal body and functions to brace the perineum against the downward pressure from the superior pelvic cavity. It has connections with the fascia from the levator ani and obturator internus muscles.

The bulbocavernosus extends from the central tendon and inferior fascia of the urogenital diaphragm anteriorly to the suspensory ligament of the clitoris and is a constrictor of the introitus; it is sometimes referred to as the sphincter vagina (Fig. 4-1).

The deep tranverse perineal muscle and a portion of the sphincter urethrae are found in the deeper layer and are referred to as the urogenital diaphragm. Separating and surrounding the muscular layers are fascial layers. Fascia plays an important role in the pelvic floor as it ensheaths the muscles and gives rise to most of the origins and insertions of those muscles.[18] The fascial layer also ensheaths the pudendal nerve and accompanying vessels. Disturbances in the fascia can cause pain, muscle spasm, decreased range of motion, vasomotor changes, sweating, and weakness. Past surgical intervention and stretching and tearing during childbirth may damage fascial tissues.

Round ligament

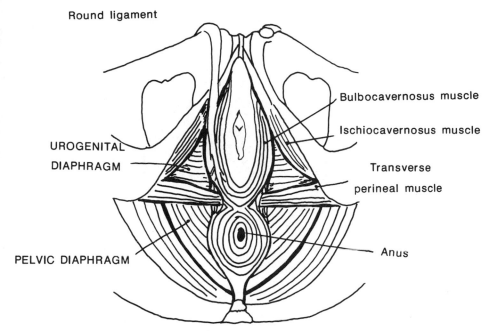

Bulbocavernosus muscle

Ischiocavernosus muscle

UROGENITAL

DIAPHRAGM

Transverse

perineal muscle

PELVIC DIAPHRAGM

Anus

Fig. 4-1.   Female pelvic diaphragm, inferior view.

Pelvic Diaphragm

Deep to the urogenital diaphragm is the pelvic diaphragm, composed of the levator ani muscles. The pelvic diaphragm extends from the pubis to the coccyx and functions in part to hold the bladder base and bladder neck in an intra-abdominal position, a position vital to the maintenance of continence. If weakness exists in the diaphragm, its supportive role is lost: the bladder base will drop into the extra-abdominal space and the crucial urethrovesical junction will be altered.[19] Increases in intra-abdominal pressure will force the bladder neck open rather than closed, and leakage will occur.

The levator ani are three composite muscles named according to their location: the pubococcygeus, the iliococcygeus, and the ischiococcygeus (coccygeus).[20] The muscles join in the midline to form a sling extending from the pubic bone in front to the coccyx behind, leaving gaps for the passage of the urethra, vagina, and rectum. The muscles arise from both sides of the posterior aspect of the os pubis (lateral to the symphysis) and from the obturator internus fascia. The most posterior fibers are inserted onto the last two coccyx segments and to the tendinous area of the perineum between coccyx and anus. The middle fibers interdigitate with the rectal sphincter while the anterior fibers interdigitate with the superficial perineal muscles (Fig. 4-2).

The pubococcygeus (the anterior portion of the levator ani) is the major muscle in the pelvic floor. This muscle supports pelvic viscera, generates

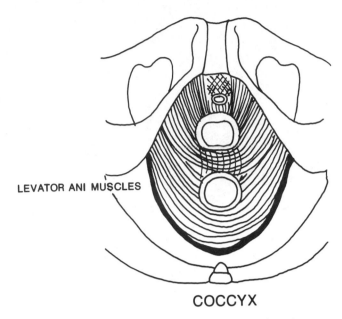

LEVATOR ANI MUSCLES

COCCYX

Fig. 4-2.   Female pelvic diaphragm, superior view.

midsphincteric control of the urethra and bowel, and is responsible for continence, for tone of the vaginal walls, and for normal sexual functioning.[8,9,18,20] No fibrous connections are present between the pubococcygeus and the urethra, yet this muscle provides an occlusive force by fascial connection and anatomic proximity.[20] Some authors consider the levator ani secondary to the fascia and ligaments as primary support of the uterus and vaginal walls.[21,22]

Pelvic floor exercises (Kegel exercises) are directed toward the pelvic diaphragm and are designed to strengthen and tone the pubococcygeus muscle. In actuality, however, voluntary contraction elicits a response in both the urogenital and pelvic diaphragms, thereby approximating the pubis and the coccyx and drawing the perineum inward.

The pubococcygeus muscle can be palpated 3 to 5 cm from the introitus[13,17] through the lateral walls of the vagina. Heardman points out that fascial connections are present between the levator ani and the sacroiliac ligaments, obturator internus, piriformis, biceps femoris, and semitendinosus muscles.[23]

Zacharin's comparative cadaver study on the quality of the levator ani muscles in western and eastern women demonstrates the presence in eastern women of greater muscle bulk, stronger support at the region of the bladder neck, more mobility, less deterioration of the muscle with age, and the ability to withstand greater intra-abdominal pressure. He attributes the differences to squatting, diet, genetics, and physical work.[24]

The triangular ischiococcygeus (coccygeus) muscle interdigitates with the sacrospinous ligament, the lower sacrum, and the upper coccyx. In its entirety, the pelvic diaphragm, containing the levator ani, forms a sling that can approximate the coccyx toward the symphysis pubis.[20] Not only do these muscles have the potential to decrease the urethral, vaginal, and rectal canals, but they can decrease the anteroposterior relationships of the bony ring; and some authors believe that they can change the angle of the sacrum to the lumbar spine.

Urinary System

The lower urinary system consists of the bladder, the urethra, and the internal and external sphincters. The urethra pierces the pelvic and urogenital diaphragms and the urogenital triangle. A major portion of the system, including the bladder base and neck, lies superior to the pelvic diaphragm in the intra-abdominal space (Fig. 4-3). Support for the structures, maintenance of the urethrovesical angle, and occlusive pressure on the urethra—all vital components for urinary continence—are provided by the pelvic diaphragm, the endopelvic fascia, the urogenital diaphragm and triangle, the pubourethral ligaments, and the pubocervical fascia.[25]

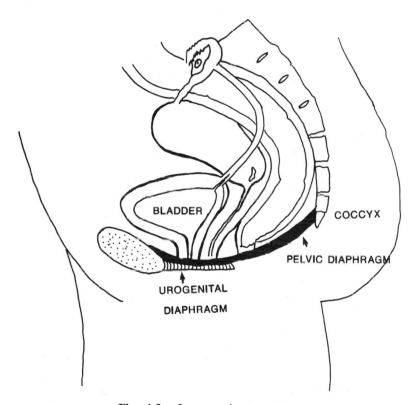

Fig. 4-3. Lower urinary system.

Micturition represents a complex series of integrated central nervous system reflexes involving the lower urinary system, the pelvic floor and abdominal musculature, the spinal cord, the brain stem, and the cerebral cortex.[26]

Continence is based on the principle that urethral resistance must be greater than the intravesical pressure. Urethral resistance requires the following:

1. A competent bladder neck supported by the pubourethral ligaments, pubocervical fascia, and the levator ani muscle platform
2. An intrinsic urethral mechanism
3. An intact external sphincter
4. An intact pelvic floor
5. Intra-abdominal pressure
6. An intact vascular content in and around the urethra[25-27]

Seventy percent of cases of incontinence are caused by bladder outlet dysfunction. In addition to adequate urethral resistance, continence requires that the detrusor and the trigone muscles of the bladder contract at the correct times in the correct sequence. Thus, the factors maintaining continence involve inert mechanisms related to the shape and anatomic structure of the bladder neck and active mechanisms which depend on activity of the muscles in or surrounding the bladder and urethra[25].

The bladder passively collects and actively expels urine. The urethra functions as an outlet or valve. During the filling phase, unconscious cortical control inhibition, mediated from the basal ganglia, suppresses the proprioceptive afferent impulses from stretch receptors in the detrusor. These impulses pass through the second, third, and fourth sacral segments of the spinal cord. As the volume in the bladder increases, impulses are relayed by way of the spinothalamic tracts to the cerebral cortex and the need to void is brought to the conscious level.[26-28]

The cortex inhibits voiding until the woman decides that conditions are socially acceptable for it. This period of time is called the postponement phase. If the postponment phase must be extended, surrounding muscles voluntarily contract to assist in increasing urethral resistance. The end of the postponment phase finds the urethral sphincter mechanism relaxing for 3 to 5 seconds, after which the detrusor contracts. These actions combine to cause intravesical pressure to rise above urethral pressure. Voiding starts once the urethral closure pressure has dropped to zero. Relaxation of pelvic floor musculature is necessary to allow descent of the bladder base and opening of the outlet neck.[25,26]

Under normal conditions, increases in intra-abdominal pressure (cough, sneeze, physical activity) elicits a reflex contraction of the pelvic diaphragm which aids in urethral resistance.[28] The pubourethral ligaments and surrounding fascia support the urethra so as to transmit abrupt increases in intra-abdominal pressure equally to the bladder and upper one-third of the urethra

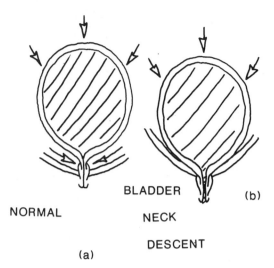

Fig. 4-4. The effect of intra-abdominal pressure on the urethra. (**A**) Normal, (**B**) bladder neck descended. (Redrawn from Powell P: Incontinence: function, dysfunction, and investigation. Physiotherapy 69:105, 1983.)

BLADDER (b)

NORMAL NECK

DESCENT

(a)

and thus prevent leakage (Fig. 4-4A) Disruption of the pubourethral ligaments and pubocervical fascia, which attach to either side of the posterior one-third of the urethra and provide support for the urethrovesical junction, may result in incontinence or prolapse[79] (Fig. 4-4B).

DYSFUNCTIONS: DEFINITION AND ASSESSMENT

Weakness of the musculature or supporting structures of the pelvic floor results in laxity. Incontinence and/or prolapse of the pelvic organs are the most common results of laxity.

Laxity: Incontinence

Incontinence, as defined by the International Continence Society, is the loss of urine at any time unacceptable to the individual.[30] Four categories of incontinence are given: stress, urge, reflex, and overflow.

Stress Incontinence

Stress incontinence is the involuntary loss of urine that occurs following a sudden rise in intra-abdominal pressure brought on by coughing, sneezing, straining, laughing, or other physical activities.[30] In this condition the urethral closure pressure is less than the intravesical pressure, and leakage occurs. Factors that cause stress incontinence include the following:

1. Abrupt fetal movements and mechanical pressure on the bladder
2. Trauma to supporting structures of the bladder and urethra at childbirth
3. Congenital weakness of the supporting structures
4. Obesity[31]
5. Elevated intra-abdominal pressure on the pelvic floor musculature from chronic cough[32]
6. Neurologic disorders affecting the outlet reflexes and musculature[3,26,32]

Partial denervation, urethral adhesions, and loss of elasticity of the tissues from prior surgeries have been cited in conditions of incontinence.[4,5,7] Also contributing to the condition are cigarette smoking, excessive coffee, tea and diuretics consumption,[27] chronic straining, repeated heavy lifting,[24] and traumatic fracture of the pelvis accompanied by rupture of the posterior urethra.[33]

The single most important variable in stress incontinence which can affect nulliparous as well as multiparous women is weakness of the pelvic floor muscles.[25] Kegel reported that 100 percent of clients with stress incontinence had some degree of difficulty contracting the levator ani muscles.[4] A survey of women attending gynecologic clinics in Australia, Canada, and England revealed that 30 percent were troubled by stress incontinence and 40 percent of all clients could not voluntarily contract the pelvic diaphragm.[34] Beck reported that for 64 percent of women with stress incontinence onset occurs during pregnancy (Table 4-1) and that half remain incontinent into the postpartum period. He reported that stress incontinence becomes progressive with subsequent pregnancies and that the incidence of stress incontinence increases with the gravid state.[34]

Assessment. Medical management of the client having stress incontinence and laxity of the pelvic musculature varies greatly. Some clients may have sought help only to be told that incontinence is a common unavoidable outcome of childbirth and that they must "grin and bear it until surgery is warranted."[1] In other cases, the client may seek out the physical therapist after multiple unsuccessful attempts with medications and surgeries.[35,36]

Correct management of the condition of laxity and stress incontinence is based on careful and thorough evaluation, with the physical therapist as an integral part of the health care team that may include a urologist, a gynecol-

Table 4-1. Time of Onset of Stress Incontinence [SI] in 1,000 Random Cases

	No. Cases	% SI Cases
During pregnancy	202	64.5
During puerperium	44	14.1
In nulligravid state	43	13.7
After menopause	8	2.6
Miscellaneous	16	5.1

(Modified from Beck R, Hsu N: Pregnancy, childbirth, and the menopause related to the development of stress incontinence. Am J Obstet Gynecol 91:820, 1963.)

ogist, an obstetrician, or a midwife. The author recommends that the physical therapist work in conjunction with other health care professionals so that an accurate diagnosis can be confirmed.

Urodynamic evaluation tests, such as a urethral pressure profile, give objective baseline measurements of the urethral closure pressure along its entire length. In response to increased intra-abdominal pressure, the woman with stress incontinence demonstrates decreased rather than increased pressures. A urodynamic stress test measures the ability of the urethrovesical junction to counter intra-abdominal pressures in a variety of positions and assists in confirming the type of incontinence.[25] Radiographs rule out anterior pelvic fractures as a source of pain and confirm perineal descent.[33,36,37] Electromyography of the external sphincters and nerve conduction studies of the musculature confirm or rule out neurologic involvement[38] and guide the therapist in treatment planning. Additionally, these objective assessments aid the clinician in evaluating intervention outcomes.

Assessment of the client by the physical therapist should begin with a detailed history. Questions regarding prior similar episodes may point to a historical incontinence that was merely aggravated by childbirth. Birthing history, onset of symptoms, prior medical intervention, and surgical and episiotomy repair should be discussed. Repeated lifting, particularly of the newborn, may contribute to the problem of incontinence. Exploring family dynamics and the client's feelings about her condition will reveal the depth of the problem and uncover assets that may be used in treatment. An evaluation form that contains relevant questions will benefit the therapist in this portion of the evaluation (Fig. 4-5).

A musculoskeletal evaluation is indicated for all clients with urogenital dysfunction, and the reader is referred to Chapters 2 and 3 of this text for specific tests and methods. The external structural examination focuses on the abdomen, thorax, pelvis, and lower quadrant. An examination for the presence of a diastasis recti and an active and passive assessment of the lumbar, lumbosacral, sacroiliac, femoral, and symphysis pubic joints is necessary. Postural changes are common in clients with chronic urogenital dysfunction. Abnormal muscle alignment may lead to secondary abnormal joint alignment. The abdominal and perineal regions should be checked for scars, tone, symmetry, and tenderness. Manual muscle testing of the abdomen, back, and lower extremities is important to detect weakness and asymmetry. The level of prolapse of the bladder, rectum, and uterus, and abnormalities of tone and symmetry of the pelvic floor musculature are determined by internal examination. The pubococcygeus muscle can be palpated 3 to 5 cm from the introitus through the lateral walls of the vagina.[13,17] Upon voluntary contraction, the fibers should approximate and provide an occlusive force on the walls.[39] A healthy muscle has a strong occlusive force and a palpatory thickness of three finger widths, whereas an atrophied muscle will be as thin as a pencil.[13] Unilateral weakness will often present, depending on the birthing conditions.[10] Palpation and voluntary contraction are an important step in teaching the client awareness and in isolating the function of the pubococcygeus muscle.

Name: _____ Age: _____ Ht: _____ Wt: _____
Occupation: _____ Years at Occupation: _____
Chief Complaint: _____
Onset of Symptoms: _____
Medical History: _____
Obstetric and Gynecological History: _____
_____

Medical Personnel Seen: _____
Medications/Birth Control: _____
Birthing History: (Date, Type of Delivery, Duration of Stages, Wt. Newborn) _
_____
_____
_____

Other Conditions: Infections ___ Pain ___ Allergies ___ Cough ___ Smoking ___
Weight Gain ___ Weight Loss ___ Falling Out Feeling ___
Incontinence Pattern: Time of Day ___ Number of Times/Day ___ Activities ___
Positions ___ Fluid Intake _____
Stress Incontinence + Unstable Bladder _____
Stress Incontinence: Mild (Occasional) ___ Moderate (Daily ___ Severe (3x) ___
Vaginal Prolapse: Cystocele ___ Rectocele ___ Uterine Prolapse ___
Perineometer Reading: Supine Rest ___ Contracted ___
                      Hooklying Rest ___ Contracted ___
Digital Examination: _____
Other Findings: _____
_____

Fig. 4-5. Assessment chart.

The Kegel perineometer (Fig. 4-6) is a pneumatic device introduced thirty years ago for assessment and treatment of pelvic floor musculature. Relatively simple in design, with a cylindrical rubber vaginal chamber and numbered gauge,[4] the perineometer is inserted by the client and registers intravaginal pressure from 0 to 100 mmHg upon contraction of the pelvic diaphragm. Clients with stress incontinence and weakened musculature register lower values than women without dysfunction.[5,6,12,13] Levitt found that continent women of ages 20 to 40 having 1 to 2 children registered differences from 5 to 15 mmHg between the resting and contractile states when assessed by the perineometer.[40] Investigators using the perineometer for assessment conclude that parity decreases the woman's capacity to voluntarily contract the pelvic diaphragm.[13,40]

Unless taught correctly, clients attempt to use gluteal, adductor, and abdominal muscle substitutions and this distorts the perineometer output. Varying the position of the perineometer can influence output by up to 20 mmHg. Other limitations include lack of fit to individual clients,[40] fluttering of the gauge,[41] lack of permanent record, and the wearing down of the resistance chamber of the perineometer over time. Despite limitations, this device offers

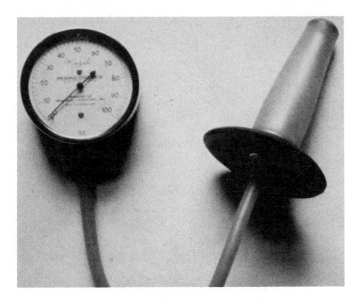

Fig. 4-6.   Kegel perineometer.

the client a means for proprioceptive input during instruction of Kegel exercises as well as visible feedback and a means for resistive isometric exercising of the pelvic diaphragm musculature (Fig. 4-7). Stoddard[42] improved the perineometer by individualizing the fit of the perineometer to the subject by means of an inflatable catheter (Fig. 4-8).

The "electronic perineometer" (Fig. 4-9) was developed for surface electrode (EMG) assessment of the pubococcygeus muscle and for biofeedback training of pelvic floor laxity and tension. The electronic perineometer is versatile, portable, and adaptable to many forms of recording instruments. Studies testing the reliability and validity of the electronic perineometer have yet to be published.

Urge Incontinence

Urge or frequency incontinence is the involuntary loss of urine associated with a strong and urgent desire to void which overcomes the voluntary capacity to inhibit bladder function.[27] In this condition the detrusor contracts at lower filling volumes and overrides the postponement phase. The condition affects 10 to 15 percent of the population.[5] An intact distal urethral mechanism can compensate, but is often weakened in pregnancy, prolapse, and aging.[26] Possible reasons for frequency incontinence include increased stimulation of the detrusor due to infection or caffeine, urinary tumor, deficient inhibition of bladder function, and fear of leaking.[27] Harrison[18] reports 30 percent of

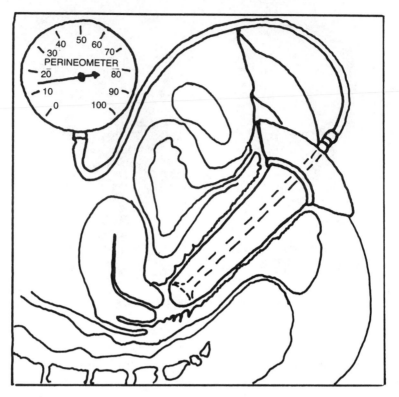

Fig. 4-7.   Kegel perineometer. (Redrawn from Kegel A: Progressive resistance exercise in functional restoration of perineal muscles. Am J Obstet Gynecol 56:238, 1948.)

physical therapy referrals for treatment of incontinence are of the urge or frequency classification.

Assessment.   Laboratory tests to determine the source and type of infection or irritant are a necessary step prior to physical therapy intervention. Cystometric measurements during the filling phase assess the pressure volume relationships in the bladder and urethra[36] and distinguish urge from stress incontinence.[25] The physical therapy evaluation should include questions regarding fluid intake. Clients often try to manage their incontinence by restriction of fluids, which can provoke dehydration. Evaluation guidelines outlined in the previous section are applicable for these clients.

Reflex Incontinence

Reflex incontinence involves interruption of the afferent and efferent responses between the spinal cord and the bladder. This type of incontinence is typically seen with progressive neurologic diseases. Physical therapy interven-

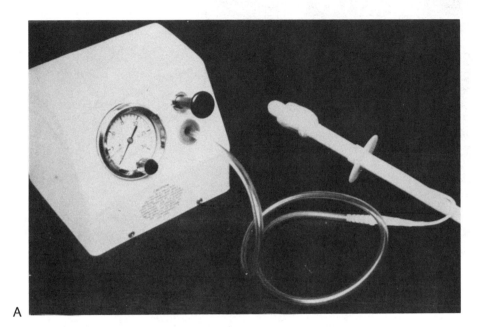

A

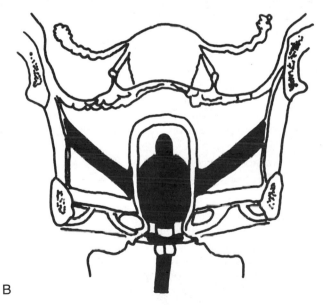

B

Fig. 4-8. **(A)** Stoddard perineometer. **(B)** Sagittal section of pelvis showing lateral view of catheter.

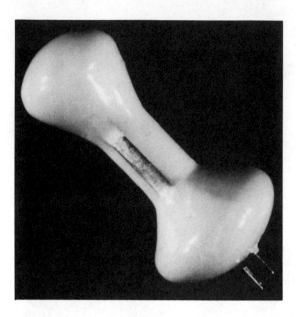

Fig. 4-9. Electronic perineometer. (Courtesy of Biotechnologies, Inc., Strafford, PA.)

tion focuses on clothing and environment modifications. Assessment of these clients should be referred to other medical personnel.

Overflow Incontinence

Overflow incontinence occurs with failure of the bladder to contract or with stricture of the urethral outlet, causing an inability to void appropriately. Detrusor incompetence of neurologic origin may prevent contraction. Pelvic floor tension or presence of a large cystocele may cause blockage of the outlet.[6,39] Accurate assessment of the client necessitates consultation with other medical personnel, and physical therapy intervention may commence following surgical repair of the cystocele. Assessment for pelvic floor tension will be discussed in a later section.

Laxity Causing Prolapse

Prolapse of the bladder (cystocele), urethra (urethrocele), rectum (rectocele), and uterus (uterine prolapse) may or may not accompany conditions of incontinence. Kegel[5] reported that 30 percent of the clients he saw with stress incontinence also had cystoceles. Of 46 patients studied by Maly for treatment of stress incontinence, 36 had first degree cystoceles. Of those 36 women, 22 had undergone at least one surgical repair operation.[7] Rectocele and/or cystocele occur in 1/10,000 pregnancies. Prolonged labor, bearing down before full dilation, laceration of the lower genital tract, and forceful delivery of the placenta are all consequences of childbirth which may lead to prolapse.[43] Complications from vaginal surgeries may also involve denervation of the pudendal nerve,[44] while abdominal surgeries can injure the hypogastric nerves, affecting innervation to the levator ani muscles and the external anal sphincter.[18,44]

Descent of the bladder through the pubocervical fascia and into the anterior vaginal wall is termed a cystocele.[45] Clients report symptoms of low backache pain, discomfort in the pelvis, difficulty in voiding, a feeling of a lump in the vaginal wall, and conditions of stress incontinence. A urethrocele is the herniation of the paravaginal fascia under the urethra, with descent of the urethra and, occasionally the uterus and cervix due to loss of support from the pubocervical and pubo-urethral ligaments. Uterine prolapse or descent of the uterus into the vaginal canal may occur with loss of support from the lateral cervical (Mackenrodt) ligament following vaginal or abdominal hysterectomy. Descent of the uterus is subjectively categorized in three degrees of severity. In a third degree prolapse, the uterus may be palpated at the opening of the introitus (Fig. 4-10). Clients complain of a falling out feeling and discomfort during sexual activities.

A herniation of the investing fascia of the posterior part of the vagina is

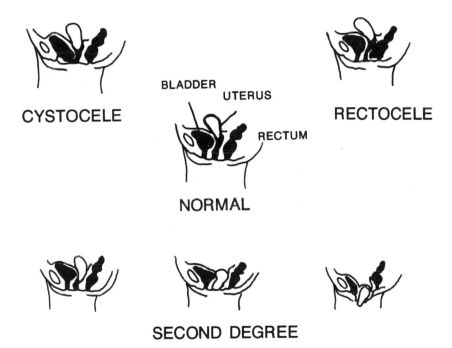

CYSTOCELE

BLADDER UTERUS

RECTUM

RECTOCELE

NORMAL

SECOND DEGREE

FIRST DEGREE   **THIRD DEGREE**

Fig. 4-10. Uterine prolapse. (Modified from Moore, KL: Clinical Oriented Anatomy. 2nd Ed. © 1985 The Williams & Wilkins Co., Baltimore.)

termed an enterocele, and may follow operations for colposuspension or hysterectomy. A rectocele is a herniation of the anterior rectal wall through the relaxed or ruptured vaginal fascia and rectovaginal septum. The supports are weakened from congenital abnormalities of the supporting structures, prolonged childbirth, or menopause. The colon bulges into the posterior wall of the vagina. Clients report difficulty or pain with defecation, low back pain, and pain or discomfort in the pelvis.

Assessment. The patient's reporting a long second stage of delivery may alert the therapist to the possibility of a prolapse. An internal examination, with instruction to the client to bear down and cough, will confirm the bulging in the anterior or posterior wall. Assessment by palpation of the pubococcygeus muscle, perineometer assessment, and musculoskeletal evaluation are advised.

DYSFUNCTION: DEFINITION AND ASSESSMENT
Excessive Tension

Following delivery, women often suffer postpartum episiotomy complications of pain, urethral disruption, scarring, and adhesions of the perineal tissues. Sacral torsions from birthing positions, innominate slips and rotations, and pubic symphysis separations lead to abnormal stresses of the connecting levator ani muscles of the pelvic diaphragm.

A condition that involves spasm and tenderness of the levator ani muscles has been termed "levator syndrome".[45-47] The client reports pain, pressure, and discomfort in the rectum, vagina, perirectal area, thighs, gluteal, or low back regions lasting from minutes to days, unrelated to defecation. Probable causes for the symptoms include neurologic abnormalities in the lumbosacral spine, pelvic malignancy, trauma, perirectal abscesses, anal fissures, prior surgeries, inflammation, and excessive anxiety.[45-47]

Urodynamic assessment of clients with "urethral syndrome" reveals an inability to relax the urethral sphincter and the muscles surrounding the urethra. Clients typically complain of low back pain, perineal pressure, unrelieved pelvic pressure, pain after bladder emptying, and dyspareunia.[15] Trauma from childbirth with tearing and scar formation, episiotomies, emotional stress, sexual abuse, infections, and prior surgical procedures are cited as probable causes. Chronic increased tension in the levator ani muscles contributes to frequent urinary tract infections.[48]

Episiotomies are the second most common surgical procedure performed in the United States, second only to cutting of the umbilical cord.[49] Pain can be severe in 60 percent of women undergoing the procedure, with dyspareunia experienced by 20 percent for up to 3 months after the episiotomy.[49] A recent study suggests that one year postpartum, perineal muscle function had not been preserved by prophylactic episiotomies. Regardless of the degree of perineal trauma, the factor which had the greatest significance relative to outcome was regular exercise.[50]

"Tension myalgia" refers to pain in the pelvic floor muscles, rectum, low back, and pelvis. The client suffers from dyspareunia, constipation, and impaired daily function.[35] Diagnosis is usually obscured by multiple and vague complaints. The general examination, x-ray, neurologic, orthopedic, and routine laboratory tests often are negative. An accurate diagnosis, therefore, must include examination of the pelvic musculature by palpation. These techniques are described in detail by Thiele.[17] Too often, misdiagnosis leads to incorrect and fruitless treatments for low back strain, lumbar disc herniation, and degenerative disc disease in the lumbar spine. According to Sim,[51] tension myalgia can be caused by repetitive muscular stresses on the pelvis in athletics and by activities that involve frequent increases in intra-abdominal pressure. This problem can be caused by habitual contraction of the pelvic floor musculature in response to pain arising anywhere in the lumbosacral spinal column, sacroiliac joint, coccyx, perineum, or hips. When the muscle tension involves the sacrospinous or sacrotubrous ligaments, pain can be referred to the back or leg.

Assessment. Assessment of the client with excessive tension must include a detailed history, observation, manual examination, and perineometer evaluation. Questions specific to episiotomy repair and rehabilitation often yield accounts of infected stitches, abscesses, fissures, poor healing, decreased sensation, and pain with intercourse. Tightening of the vaginal introitus by the "extra stitch" or "husband's knot" may be a source of reflexive spasm and tenderness of the pubococcygeus muscle. Lack of mobility in the sutured region, tenderness medial to the ischial spines, and inability to release the introitus are common findings.

Musculoskeletal evaluation is essential for these conditions, as the positioning of the sacrum, coccyx, and ilium will cause stress to the pelvic diaphragm musculature. Imbalances of the abdominal and back musculature are likely causes of a contracted and tender levator ani muscle and should be thoroughly evaluated. Assessment of the pelvic musculature using the electronic perineometer is preferred to the Kegel perineometer in conditions of abnormally high resting tonus of the muscle. A summary of the common symptoms of clients with excessive tension in the pelvic diaphragm is found in Table 4-2.

TREATMENT PLANNING

Ideally, the process of goal setting for a client is a coordinated effort involving all members of the health care team, including the client. If the therapist is not functioning in a setting where involvement of many disciplines is a viable approach, the therapist can progress through the treatment planning process according to his or her role in the client's care.

Having collected data from the evaluation process, which should include perineometer assessment, manual examination, and possibly urodynamic assessment, the therapist establishes a prioritized list of problems and client assets which focus on the positive data elicited from the evaluation process.

Table 4-2. Symptoms and Aggravating Factors
in Patients with Excessive Tension

Symptoms
    Pain in low back, rectum, perirectal area, vaginal, gluteal
      area, thighs
    Pain at rest
    Unilateral or bilateral leg pain
    Pressure in pelvic region
    Spasm, tenderness in levator ani muscles, lower
      extremity adductors
    Constipation
    Dyspareunia
    Joint malalignment in sacroliliac, lumbosacral, symphysis
      pubis, coccygeal joints
Factors that aggravate symptoms
    Sitting for more than one-half hour
    Stress
    Physical activity/lifting
    Standing for more than one-half hour
    Sexual intercourse
    Chronic cough

From this list, long term and short term goals are established with measurable, time-defined behavioral objectives to be demonstrated by the client. In cases of laxity, these goals will most often include the following:

    Promotion of homeostasis of the autonomic nervous system
    Increased perineometer readings
    Promotion of "dry" conditions with physical activity
    Promotion of reduced cystocele size

The therapist develops strategies with specific treatment procedures to address individual goals. This plan is implemented by treating the client. During each session, ongoing and formal reevaluation testing takes place to assess intervention outcome and attainment of goals.

TREATMENT PROCEDURES

Promoting homeostasis of the autonomic nervous system is the first objective of treatment and is based upon assessment of the client's current status. Clients are typically embarrassed, worried, or angry about their condition. Thus, parasympathetic input may assist in homeostatic balancing. Often, history taking and calm discussion in a quiet environment may be sufficient. Neutral warmth, relaxation exercises, and calming visualizations have therapeutic value and improve the receptivity of the client to the intervention that follows.

Over 60 different procedures are available for correction of urinary incontinence. Surgical intervention is suggested for treatment of second and third degree cystocele, rectocele, and prolapse of the uterus.[4,5,13] Complications which can occur include wound infection, incisional hernias, urinary retention, urinary tract infections, partial denervation, adhesions, decreased sensation, and voiding difficulties.[14] Thus, the physical therapist may treat the client for symptoms arising from surgery. Drug therapy is appropriate for clients with detrusor instability, urethral constricture, inconclusive diagnoses, and as an adjunct to therapy.[27,43,52]

In 1948, Kegel published an exercise prescription for restoration of lax or atrophied perineal muscles and for treatment of first degree cystocele and rectocele.[5] Kegel's pelvic floor exercises are one part of an exercise prescription individually tailored to the patient with urogenital dysfunction. Exercises to strengthen and balance abdominal, back, and lower quadrant musculature are vital to the rehabilitation program and should therefore be included. The aim of pelvic floor exercise is to counter any descent of the pelvic viscera, thereby restoring the natural anatomic relationships of the structures.[4,39] Patients are instructed to contract the pubococcygeus for 20 minutes 3 times a day with the perineometer in place for awareness and resistance. Three hundred additional contractions without the perineometer in place were performed throughout the day. The lithotomy position was recommended, and contractions by the gluteal, abdominal, and adductor muscles were discouraged. Complete relief from stress incontinence could be expected in 6 to 8 weeks.[4,5,10]

Millard[52] describes increased passive tonus of both the smooth and striated components of the pelvic contents as a goal of these exercises. With active contraction of the pelvic diaphragm muscles, all supportive and sphincteric structures of the pelvis work synergistically.[39] Teaching awareness of function of the pubococcygeus muscle was another goal mentioned by Kegel for his exercises.[4] One study found this lack of awareness present in 20 normal nulliparous women between 25 and 35 years of age. Of the 20, 13 could not isolate the pubococcygeus muscle without using either the gluteus maximus, adductor magnus, or external oblique muscles.[53] The benefits from Kegel exercises[4,5,10,43] have been summarized in Table 4-3. Rupture of episiotomy sutures and overstrengthening of the pelvic floor causing problems with relaxation during childbirth have been the only negative results reported from these exercises.[14]

Variations to Kegel's prescription include discontinuance of the use of the perineometer and digital instruction, decreased number of contractions to be done per day, differing positions for exercise, and contractions of all surrounding musculature as opposed to isolated contraction of the pubococcygeus muscle.[7,23,54,55] Some therapists recommend that clients isolate pubococcygeus function by interruption of voiding by active contraction.[18,20] Millard[52] advises against this form of instruction, suggesting that urinary tract infections may result as a consequence of the back-up of fluid. Clients reported improvement in symptoms of stress incontinence within 2 weeks of exercising without use of the perineometer.[40,43] Other authors cite significantly higher improvements in symptoms and urodynamic reevaluation in clients using the perineometer and exercises.[42,56,57] Burgio[58] stated emphatically that the most important aspect of the pelvic floor exercise program was biofeedback. Castleden[56] believes the success of the physical therapy program depends on the instruc-

Table 4-3. Benefits from Pelvic Floor (Kegel) Exercises

Maintenance of strength, tone, and elasticity of muscle
  and fascial tissues
Ability to release undue tension while birthing
Reduced need for episiotomy
Decreased feeling of heaviness in the pelvis
Heightened sexual response
Avoidance of pelvic problems, including urinary stress
  incontinence and prolapses
Change in position of the perineum, introitus, urethra,
  bladder neck and uterus
Increase in length and snugness of the vagina
Decrease of anterior vaginal wall (cystocele)
Improved sexual functioning
Relief from dyspareunia
Improved involution of the uterus in the early
  postpartum period
Decreased nocturia
Relief from hemorrhoidal pain
Relief from vulvar varicosities

tor's enthusiasm and knowledge and on the patient's motivation and cooperation.

Lack of patient compliance can be a major problem in rehabilitation programs related to the pelvic floor.[59] Isolated contractions of the pubococcygeus in patients with partial denervation of the pudendal and pelvic nerves may prove an impossible task, causing frustration and decreased motivation. Voss, Ionta, and Meyers recommend a lower extremity proprioceptive neuromuscular facilitation exercise pattern for rehabilitation using the principles of overflow and irradiation.[60] The pattern utilizes muscles involved with hip extension, hip adduction, and hip external rotation to facilitate a pubococcygeus contraction (Fig. 4-11). Additionally, a symmetrical pattern of the lower extremities may enable the client to better contract the pubococcygeus muscle (Fig. 4-12). Studies have demonstrated overflow and irradiation to the ipsilateral and contralateral limbs, with greatest electromyographic activity in muscles that are required to stabilize the body.[61] The pubococcygeus muscle is considered a stabilizing muscle by some. Heardman's definitive text on physical therapy in obstetrics describes a series of exercises that includes isolation of the pubococcygeus, along with simultaneous contractions of the abdominal, gluteal, and adductor muscles. She recommends that strengthening of the pelvic floor include strengthening of the obturatus internus, with squatting as the position that best utilizes that muscle as an abductor and lateral rotator of the hip.[23]

ELECTRICAL STIMULATION

The successful treatment of stress incontinence and pelvic laxity by isometric contractions of the pubococcygeus muscle depends to a great extent on patient cooperation and motivation. If the exercises are not performed, improvement in the contractile abilities of the muscle will not be seen.[40]

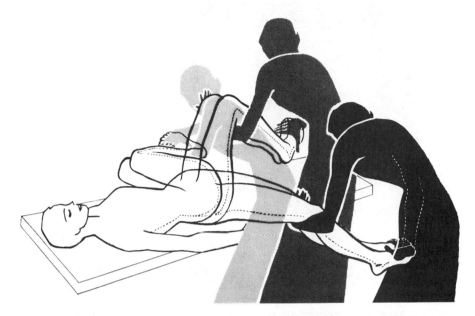

Fig. 4-11. Diagonal lower extremity pattern. (Voss D, Ionta M, Myers B. Proprioceptive neuromuscular facilitation. 3rd Ed. Harper & Row, Philadelphia, 1986.)

Electric stimulation involving a constant, pulsed current can be delivered
by a vaginal or rectal electrode to stimulate the muscles of the pelvic floor as an
adjunct to exercises or as a means to get better patient compliance.

A hand-held, battery operated, high volt galvanic stimulator (Vagette 76)
can be used as a passive exerciser in the treatment of pelvic floor laxity (Fig.
4-13). Pubococcygeal muscle strength improved significantly with this stimulation when assessed by the Kegel perineometer. Muscle strength improved even
more when stimulation was combined with a program of Kegel exercises.[59]

Eight clients had complete symptomatic relief and a return to normal
urodynamic pressures following faradic stimulation under anaesthesia.[62]
Square wave electrotherapy and daily Kegel exercises produced decreased
numbers of incontinent episodes in over 90 percent of clients investigated[63].
Recovery lasted up to 4 months from 1 application of electric stimulation with
internal electrodes,[64] and 3 months following faradic stimulation.[32] Some
investigators have questioned the benefits of electric stimulation on changing
urethral pressure measurements; Kegel exercises were found to be effective,
but electric stimulation had no additional effect. Awareness training of the
pubococcygeus muscle and use of a biofeedback device such as a perineometer
were the major factors for successful treatment outcomes.[2]

Krauss and Lilien recommend transcutaneous electric nerve stimulation to
the perineal region to improve symptoms of stress incontinence.[65] Interferential therapy was used successfully with women having partially denervated

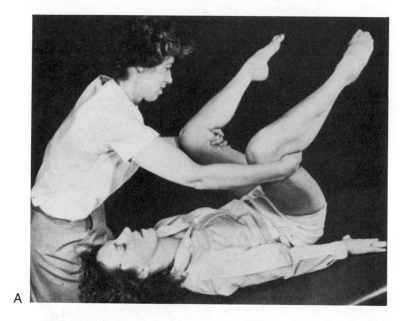

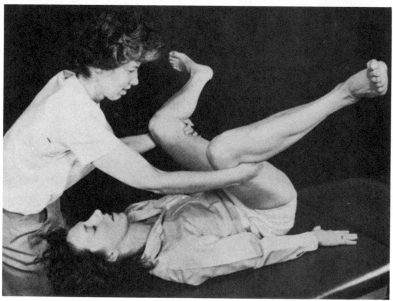

Fig. 4-12.   (A,B) Lower extremity bilateral symmetrical D2 extension pattern. (Voss D, Ionta M, Myers B: Proprioceptive neuromuscular facilitation. 3rd Ed. Harper & Row, Philadelphia, 1986.)

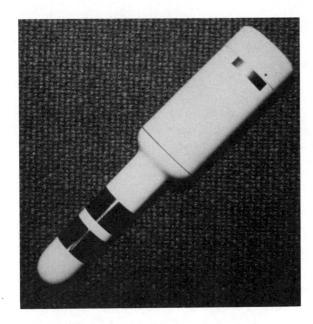

Fig. 4-13. Vagette 76. (Courtesy of Interactive Medical Technologies, Inc., Carson, CA.)

pudendal nerves, disuse atrophy, damage to sphincter muscles, and deterioration of the mucosal lining of the vagina[1,55]. Interferential therapy reduced incontinence, hemorrhoidal pain, and abdominal pain in 91 percent of clients in 12 treatments.[1]

TREATMENT: EXCESSIVE TENSION

Clients with excessive tension in the pelvic diaphragm report primary symptoms of pain, tenderness, impaired sexual activities, micturition, and defecation. Frequent urinary and vaginal infections, joint pain, and impaired sitting, standing, and physical activities are common.

The primary goals for clients with levator syndrome, urethral syndrome, or tension myalgia include the following:

Promotion of homeostasis of the autonomic nervous system
Normalization of tone in the pelvic diaphragm
Restoration of proper joint alignment and function
Muscle reeducation
Promotion of positive self-imaging

Interdisciplinary team coordination with medical personnel to diagnose and treat likely primary causes is vital to successful management. Large cystoceles/rectoceles, infections, anal fissures, perineal abscesses, and inflamed tissues must be treated. Muscle relaxants, antibiotics, anti-inflammatory medication, or surgery may be prescribed.[15]

Postpartum women commonly report negative changes in body image, endurance, sexuality, and feelings about intimacy. Psychotherapeutic intervention is helpful, and sexual counseling may help if problems are chronic.

Physical therapy procedures of heat, massage, manual therapy, muscle reeducation using biofeedback, and electrotherapy have proven beneficial in attainment of goals.[17,57,63] General inhibition techniques of neutral warmth, slow rhythmic rocking, and maintained pressure at the midline may assist in balancing the nervous system. Hot packs, sitz baths, and hydrotherapy increase circulation and aid in local and general relaxation. Continuous ultrasound can be applied to the perineal region using conductive gel or with the client sitting in water. Diathermy administered in the sitting or recumbent position promotes circulation.

Transverse friction massage mobilizes the episiotomy scar. As advocated by Rood, maintained pressure over tendons, specifically, medial to the ischial spines and anterior to the coccyx, may reduce tone in the levator ani muscles.

Biofeedback training with use of the electronic perineometer or Kegel's perionemeter is recommended for muscle reeducation. The relative difference between resting and contracted states can be assessed using the Kegel perineometer, but the resting state is best assessed by the electronic perineometer. Clients are taught to consciously relax the muscles of the pelvic floor and achieve lower resting values. Sustained maximal voluntary contractions

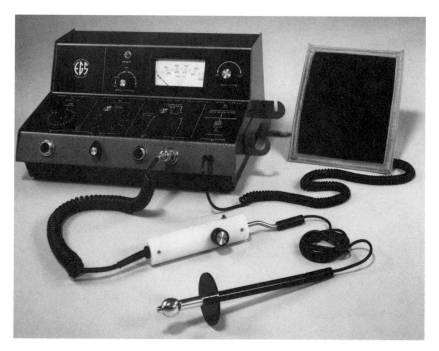

Fig. 4-14.   High volt galvanic stimulator with Sohn electrode. (Courtesy of Electro-Med Health Industries, Inc. Miami, FL.)

fatigue the levator ani muscles through golgi tendon organ mechanisms. Maly successfully treated 16 of 24 women with diagnoses of dyspareunia and vaginismus using Kegel exercises for muscle reeducation.[7] Manual therapy using the Maitland, Cyriax, Kaltenborn, or Paris technique corrects painful joint malalignments and prevents subsequent abnormal stresses to the pelvic diaphragm musculature. Abnormal sacral torsion, tilting, nutation, symphysis pubis separations, and lumbosacral, sacroiliac, and coccygeal joint changes occur as a result of birthing stresses. The clinician should be aware that hypermobility of joints exists during the prenatal and early postnatal periods and thus mobilization should be performed with caution.

Restoration of the abdominal muscles is discussed in Chapter 6. Strengthening and balancing of the abdominal, back, and hip musculature restore the normal resting tone of the pelvic diaphragm muscles. High volt electrogalvanic stimulation with a rectal probe has been successful[46–48] in treating the levator syndrome. In one study, 90 percent of the clients investigated experienced complete relief from pain for up to 6 months following 3 1-hour stimulations.[46] A vaginal probe is available from the manufacturer (Figs. 4-14, 4-15). Transcutaneous nerve stimulation applied to the perineal and sacral regions is effective in reducing pain[65]. Interferential current using anteroposterior crisscross electrode placement improves circulation and reduces pain[1,52,66] (Fig. 4-16). (For a summary of recommended treatments for dysfunction from excessive tension, see Table 4-4.)

SUMMARY

Urogenital dysfunction may arise from numerous conditions that affect the supporting structures and muscles of the pelvic floor. Childbearing and childbirth are events that may aggravate congenital problems or create problems due to multiple hormonal, biomechanical, and anatomic changes. These problems result in conditions of laxity, commonly manifested as incontinence and prolapse, and of excessive tension, manifested as pain, dyspareunia, and vaginismus. Accurate diagnosis of the conditions can only be made if a manual

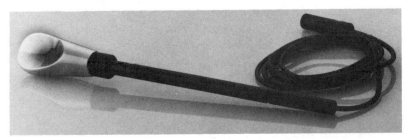

Fig. 4-15.   Vaginal electrode. (Courtesy of Electro-Med Health Industries, Inc. Miami, FL.)

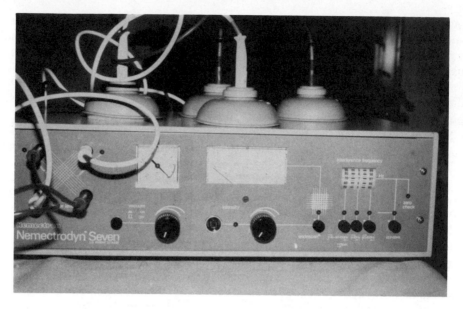

Fig. 4-16. Interferential stimulator.

examination, perineometer evaluation, and urodynamic assessment are employed along with other evaluative methods.[4,20,39,43]

Manual examination is necessary for information regarding tissue condition and functioning. Perineometer assessment is necessary for objective measurement of awareness of function, contractile abilities of the musculature, and benefits of therapeutic intervention. Urodynamic tests are a necessary and invaluable means for accurate differentiation between types of incontinence.

Patient selection is an important variable in the success of treatment.[39] Women under consideration for surgery for incontinence may improve sufficiently with physical therapy intervention of muscle reeducation, biofeedback training, electrotherapy, and education so as to make surgery unnecessary. In cases where an operation has been unsuccessful or only partially effective,

Table 4-4. Recommended Treatment for Excessive
Tension of the Pelvic Diaphragm

Rule out infection, fissure, abscess.
Administer muscle relaxants, antibiotics.
General inhibition: neutral warmth, rocking, pressure.
Apply heat using hot packs, baths, ultrasound, diathermy.
Apply friction and connective tissue massage.
Apply manual therapy.
Reeducate muscle with Kegel and therapeutic exercises.
Strengthen abdomen and back.
Provide postural instruction.
Modify tension with biofeedback, relaxation exercises.
Apply high volt galvanic stimulation.
Apply transcutaneous nerve stimulation.

physical therapy intervention may succeed. In cases where stress incontinence is accompanied by detrusor instability, results will be less satisfactory, but cystometric examinations demonstrate that pelvic floor exercises can reinforce bladder retraining. Treatments for levator syndrome, urethral syndrome, and tension myalgia have been recommended by various authors. Physical therapy procedures of heat, massage, electrotherapy, manual therapy, and muscle reeducation can be successful. Physical therapists are the most qualified health professionals to apply these treatment techniques and should be recognized as such.

Lack of compliance with the exercise prescription, poor instructional technique, and inadequate and subjective outcome assessment are problems that have plagued successful outcome. The knowledgeable physical therapist will find that the use of perineometers will improve client motivation; that thorough individualized Kegel exercise instruction will insure client understanding; and that objective evaluation tools will assist in accurate treatment reevaluation. As musculoskeletal experts, physical therapists are capable of making significant impact on clients suffering from urogenital dysfunction.

REFERENCES

1. Chirarelli P, O'Keefe D: Physiotherapy for the pelvic floor. Aust J Physiotherapy 27:4, 1981
2. Brown J: Role of the physiotherapist in obstetrics and gynecology. Physiotherapy 64:228, 1978
3. Anderson R: A neurogenic element to urinary genuine stress incontinence. Br J Obstet Gynecol 91:41, 1984
4. Kegel A: Progressive resistance exercise in the functional restoration of the perineal muscles. Am J Obstet & Gynecol 56:238, 1948
5. Kegel A, Powell T: The physiologic treatment of urinary stress incontinence. J Urol 63:808, 1950
6. Kegel A: Office treatment of genital prolapse. Curr Med Digest 7:27, 1953
7. Maly B: Rehabilitation principles in the care of gynecologic and obstetric patients. Arch Phys Med Rehabil 61:78, 1980
8. Kegel A: Sexual functions of the pubococcygeus muscle. Western Journal of Surgery, Obstetrics and Gynecology 10:521, 1952
9. Graber B, Kline-Graber G: Female orgasm: role of pubococcygeus muscle. J of Clin Psychiatry 40:348, 1979
10. Kegel A: Stress incontinence and genital relaxation. CIBA Clinical Symposium 4:35, 1952
11. Kegel A: Physiologic treatment of poor tone and function of genital muscles. Western Journal of Surgery, Obstetrics and Gynecology 57:527, 1949
12. Kegel A: Physiologic therapy for urinary stress incontinence. JAMA 146:915, 1951
13. Kegel A: Early genital relaxation. Obstet Gynecol 8:545, 1956
14. Tchou D: A descriptive study of the effects of pelvic floor exercises in the treatment of anatomical urinary stress incontinence. Unpublished thesis. Birmingham, Alabama, University of Alabama, 1986
15. Schmidt R, Tanagho E: Urethral syndrome or urinary tract infection? Urol 18:424, 1981

16. Fordney D: Dyspareunia and vaginismus. Clin Obstet Gynecol 21:205, 1978
17. Thiele G: Coccygodynia: cause and treatment. Dis Colon Rectum 6:442, 1963
18. Harrison S: Stress incontinence and the physiotherapist. Physiotherapy 69:144, 1983
19. Mikuta J, Payne F: Stress urinary incontinence in the female. Am J of Med Sci 226:647, 1953
20. Mandelstam D: The pelvic floor. Physiotherapy 64:236, 1978
21. Baden W, Walker T: Physical diagnosis in the evaluation of vaginal relaxation. Clin Obstet Gynecol 15:1055, 1972
22. Lee R: The vaginal approach to anterior vaginal relaxation. Clin Obstet Gynecol 15:1098, 1972
23. Herdman H: Physiotherapy in Obstetrics and Gynecology. E and S Livingstone Ltd., Edinburgh, 1959
24. Zacharin R: "A chinese anatomy"-The pelvic supporting tissues in the chinese and occidental female compared and contrasted. Aust N Z J Obstet Gynaec 17:1, 1977
25. Stanton S: Urethral Sphincter Incompetence. p. 169. In Stanton S [ed]: Clinical Gynecologic Urology. CV Mosby, St. Louis, 1984
26. Bent A, Ostergard D: Why women are prone to incontinence. Contemporary Ob/Gyn 1:83, 1984
27. Palmer M: Urinary Incontinence. Slack Inc., Thorofare, New Jersey, 1985
28. Powell P: Incontinence: function, dysfunction and investigation. Physiotherapy 69:105, 1983
29. Jones E: Role of active exercise in pelvic muscle physiology. Western Journal of Surgery, Obstetrics and Gynecology 58:1, 1950
30. Palmer, M: Urinary Incontinence. Slack Inc., Thorofare, New Jersey, 1985
31. Shepherd A: Management of urinary incontinence: prevention or cure. Physiotherapy 69:109, 1983
32. Schach R: Urinary stress incontinence. S Afr Med J 46:845, 1972
33. Devine P, Devine C: Posterior urethral injuries associated with pelvic injuries. Urol 20:467, 1984
34. Beck R, Hsu N: Pregnancy, childbirth and the menopause. Am J Obstet Gynecol 91:820, 1965
35. Sinaki M, Merritt J, Stillwell K: Tension myalgia of the pelvic floor. Mayo Clin Proc 52:717, 1977
36. Keighley M, Shouler P: Outlet syndrome, is there a surgical option? J Roy Soc of Med 77:553, 1984
37. Mohr M: Stress urinary incontinence: a simple practical approach to diagnosis and treatment. Am J Ger Soc 31:476, 1983
38. Hutch J, Elliott H: Electromyographic study of electrical activity in the paraurethral muscles prior to and during voiding. J Urol 99:759, 1968
39. Mandelstam D: Physiotherapy. In Stanton S [ed]: Clinical Gynecologic Urology. CV Mosby, St. Louis, 1984
40. Levitt E, Konovsky M, Freese M: Intravaginal pressure assessed by the Kegel perineometer. Arch of Sexual Behavior 8:425, 1979
41. Perry J: The vaginal myograph. Paper read to the Biofeedback Society of New England, Wakefield, Massachusettes, November 11, 1979
42. Stoddard G: Research project into the effect of pelvic floor exercises on genuine stress incontinence. Physiotherapy 69:148, 1983
43. Gordon H, Loque M: Perineal muscle function after childbirth. Lancet 2:123, 1985

44. Percy J, Neill M, Swash M: Electrophysiological study of motor nerve supply of pelvic floor. Lancet 1:16, 1981
45. Sohn N, Weinstein M, Robbins R: The levator syndrome and its treatment with high-voltage electrogalvanic stimulation. Am J Surgery 144:581, 1982
46. Oliver G, Rubin R, Salvati E: Electrogalvanic stimulation in the treatment of levator syndrome. Dis Colon Rectum 28:662, 1985
47. Nicosia J, Abcarian H: Levator syndrome. Dis Colon Rectum 28:406, 1985
48. Perry J, Whipple B: Diagnostic, therapeutic, and research applications of the vaginal myograph. Presentation at AASECT, March 6, 1980
49. Banta D, Thacker S: Benefits and risks of episiotomy. p. 80. In Kitzinger S, Simkin P [eds]: Episiotomy and the Second Stage of Labor. Pennypress, Seattle, 1986
50. Simkin P: Review of research findings. p. 109. In Kitzinger S, Simkin P [eds]: Episiotomy and the Second Stage of Labor. Pennypress, Seattle, 1986
51. Sim F, Scott S: Injuries of the pelvis and hip in athletes: anatomy and function. p. 1119. In Nicholas J, Hershman E [eds]: The Lower Extremity and Spine in Sports Medicine. CV Mosby, St. Louis, 1986
52. Millard R: The conservative management of urinary incontinence. Aust Physiotherapy Assoc Nat Ob/Gyn Group Bulletin 3:30, 1982
53. Herman H: An EMG study of the pubococcygeus muscle using a torque-EMG perineometer. Presentation at the Nat APTA Mid-Winter Conf, Orlando, Florida, February, 1985
54. Noble E: Essential Exercises For The Childbearing Year. 2nd Ed. Houghton-Mifflin, Boston, 1983
55. Wharton L: The nonoperative treatment of stress incontinence in women. J Urol 69:511, 1953
56. Castleden C, Duffin H, Mitchell E: The effect of physiotherapy on stress incontinence. Age and Aging 13:235, 1984
57. Shepherd A, Montgomery E: Treatment of genuine stress incontinence with a new perineometer. Physiotherapy 69:113, 1983
58. Burgio K, Robinson J, Engel B: The role of biofeedback in Kegel exercise training for urinary stress incontinence. Am J Obstet Gynecol 154:58, 1986
59. Scott R, Hseuh G: A clinical study of the effects of galvanic vaginal muscle stimulation in urinary stress incontinence and sexual dysfunction. Am J Obstet Gynecol 135:663, 1979
60. Voss D, Ionta M, Myers B: Proprioceptive Neuromuscular Facilitation. 3rd Ed. Harper & Row, Philadelphia, 1986
61. Markos P: Ipsilateral and contralateral effects of proprioceptive neuromuscular facilitation techniques on hip motion and electromyographic activity. Phys Ther 59:1366, 1979
62. Turner A: An appraisal of maximal faradic stimulation of pelvic muscles in the management of female urinary incontinence. Ann R Coll Surg Eng 61:441, 1979
63. Montgomery E, Shepherd A: Electrical stimulation and graded pelvic exercises for genuine stress incontinence. Physiotherapy 69:4:112, 1983
64. Plevnik S: Maximal electrical stimulation for urinary incontinence. Urol 14:638, 1979
65. Krauss D, Lilien O: Transcutaneous nerve stimulation for stress incontinence. J Urol 125:790, 1981
66. Haag W: Practical experience with interference current therapy in gynaecology. Der Frauenarzt 1:1, 1979

5 | Electrical Modalities in Obstetrics and Gynecology

Joseph Kahn

The conscientious physical therapy practitioner must apply his/her expertise to all phases of medical practice, among which should be obstetrics/gynecology (OB/GYN). This chapter may serve as a review for those already involved in this specialty, or as an introduction to an area whose full potential has yet to be realized in physical therapy practice.

Shortwave diathermy has long been known to be an effective modality for treating pelvic inflammation. Increased blood flow, analgesia, and enhanced drainage are benefits of deep heating of the pelvis in the nonacute stages.[1-4] High frequency heating of this type offers deeper penetration without superficial heating. Tissues are heated by induction (rather than by conduction, radiation or convection); the heat causes gases trapped within confined structures (e.g. blood vessels, alveoli) to expand. This phenomenon follows the traditional physical laws of Boyle and Charles relating to the relationships between gaseous volumes and temperature/pressure changes. As the gases expand, pressure against the walls of vessels results in increased lumens of the vessels, leading to greater transmission of fluids, including blood and reticuloendothelial system drainage. In 1943, R.L. Craig and H. Kraff at Lincoln Hospital in New York suggested the importance of absorption of inflammatory exudates in pelvic inflammatory diseases.[3] The mild heating and temperature elevation provide a soothing effect on the irritated nerve endings and help to increase the membrane permeability in the heated region. All of the benefits attributed to this localized heating may be obtained with shortwave diathermy. The effects of shortwave diathermy are mild and are generally distributed throughout the target tissues, since the heat generated is dependent upon the

113

density and water content of the tissues themselves. Of course, any form of heating is contra-indicated in the face of acute inflammation. Care must also be taken with medications which may affect the patient's ability to sense heat or discomfort. Profuse discharge during menses may also result from excessive heating and subsequent increased circulatory stimulation.

If effective, diathermy may be administered daily or every other day for analgesic effects and relaxation of pelvic musculature in spasm due to inflammation.

Drum-type or condenser pad techniques are equally effective in diathermy applications. Of the two, the drum units are more easily applied in most cases. With the patient supine and supported under the knees for comfort, the hinged drum is placed across the lower abdomen with sufficient towel insulation at the iliac spines to avoid overheating at those points (Fig. 5-1). With condenser pads, the abdomen is "sandwiched" between pads placed anteroposterior, even if the patient is sidelying (Fig. 5-2). Twenty minutes of mild heat will usually provide the desired analgesia. Patients sometimes report a flushed sensation and momentary vertigo when sitting up after the treatment. Allow for this orthostatic adjustment when evaluating results. Symptomatic relief is usually immediate. Additional modalities, such as electrical stimulation, may be indicated and administered following diathermy. (Electrical stimulation is covered in the next section.)

Microthermy has also been reported effective in pelvic inflammation

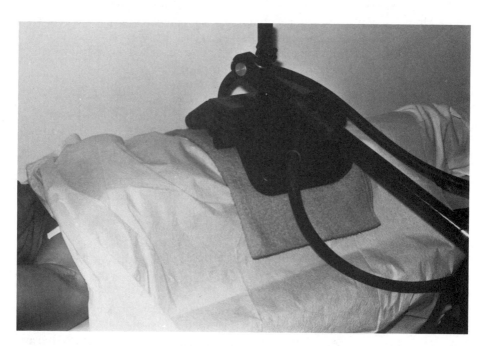

Fig. 5-1. Shortwave diathermy with induction drum across the lower abdomen, showing toweling protecting the bony prominences. (Birtcher Corp.)

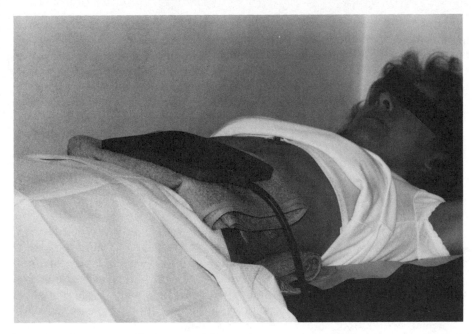

Fig. 5-2. Shortwave diathermy with condenser pads placed anteroposterior with toweling between pads and skin. (Lindquist Corp.)

management. With higher frequency microwave transmission and directed applicators, heat is more concentrated locally. Penetration is compromised by intervening layers of adipose tissue, where much of the microwave transmission is absorbed before reaching the selected target tissues. Proper applicator and power selection are determining factors with successful microthermy treatment. These factors are determined by the physical therapist at the time of administration.

The physics of microthermy differs greatly from shortwave diathermy, not only in frequency (3450 MHz versus diathermy's 12.5–45.0 MHz) and wave length (10.5–12.0 cm versus diathermy's 7, 11, and 22 m), but also in the manner of production of the effective transmission. Diathermy utilizes standard power and frequency amplification devices, (e.g., transformers, oscillators, solid state electronic components), whereas microthermy radiation results from the enhanced frequencies obtained from a magnetron, a device designed to multiply frequencies via electron acceleration. The heat produced provides the enumerated physiologic advantages within the target tissues. However, microthermy's area of influence is much smaller in volume than diathermy's. Depths of penetration vary with both modalities, depending upon intervening tissues and structures. In general, shortwave diathermy heats mildly in a greater volume while microthermy heats more intensely in a smaller volume. For example, diathermy may heat the entire lower abdominal cavity mildly; microthermy may heat just a unilateral ovarian section more intensely.

Both diathermy and microthermy are useful in the management of pelvic inflammation. Selection is usually determined by previous experience, available apparatus, and clinicians' preference. The reported results have been essentially the same. (The availability of microthermy equipment is limited at this time due to restrictions and revised regulations of the FDA.)

Few physicians are familiar with physical therapy modalities and techniques. Physical therapists should not expect specific instructions with referrals. Each clinician should be prepared to offer advice and suggested procedures when and where applicable.

ELECTRICAL STIMULATION

Electrical stimulation is frequently utilized in gynecologic conditions, with favorable results. Benefits attributed to electric stimulation include relaxation of spasmodic musculature, weight-free exercises for weakened muscles, softening of adhesions and scar tissue, reeducation of traumatized muscles with nerve damage, and aiding in the minimizing, delaying, and possible prevention of disuse atrophy. Recent information in the literature suggests increased endorphin production with electrical stimulation.[5] One of the points often overlooked is that electrical stimulation increases recruitment of fibers compared with normal motion.

A viable alternative to diathermy/microthermy during the menstrual period is mild electrical stimulation to the lower lumbar and sacral nerve roots. Stress incontinence and pelvic floor weakness have been treated by electrical stimulation for more than forty years.[6] This procedure is enjoying a current revival according to the literature and to the manufacturers of instruments for this purpose.

The mild heat produced by electric energy (Joule's Law), the consequent rise in tissue temperature, and pumping phenomena of the electrically stimulated muscles all combine to produce favorable effects without considerable increase of menstrual activity. This is because the heat produced is superficial at the electrode/skin interface and is negligible in intensity. These desired effects may include mild analgesia due to the decongestion of accrued inflammatory fluids, relaxation of myospasm, and increased circulation in the area.

Surged AC is the mode of choice, usually at a frequency of 100 Hz surged 6 to 10 times per minute and directed at the lumbar/sacral nerve roots. These parameters will produce a comfortable contraction without skin irritation. For a more generalized stimulation of the lower regions, the gluteal muscles may be included in the treatment (Fig. 5-3). Except for the gluteals, visible or palpable contractions may not be elicited; however, they are not required since the deeper muscle groups are the prime targets. Obviously, the deeper layers will receive appropriately less stimulation because of the intervening resistance. Only the reaction of the superficial gluteals will be visible. The contractions and subsequent associated contraction of deeper adjacent musculature will be

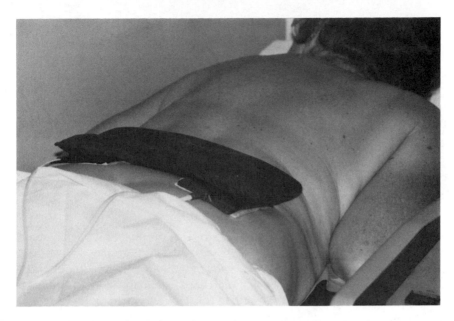

Fig. 5-3. Electrical stimulation with EMS unit; electrodes placed at paravertebral nerve roots and gluteal motor points. (Chattanooga Corp.)

obtained secondary to the gluteal stimulation and will generally cover a wider target zone.

When the condition to be treated is stress incontinence, the use of a vaginal electrode is recommended.[6-11] This specialized electrode, available through most dealers, is first warmed in water then covered with a thin layer of conductive gel and inserted into the vagina as far as possible without discomfort. A secondary electrode is placed on the anterior abdomen (suprapubic region). Tetanizing current (100 Hz AC) is recommended for the first few minutes to relax the musculature of the vaginal walls and perineum. Although the prime targets for electric stimulation with stress incontinence are weakened sphincter muscles, the adjacent musculature often displays protective spasm. The sphincter musculature may itself be in spasm. Following this brief tetanization, surged AC at 100 Hz is then administered with 6 to 10 surges per minute for 10 to 20 minutes.

If a galvanic apparatus of high voltage (i.e., 300 to 500 volts pulsed DC, microsecond pulse duration) is utilized for this purpose, only one of the two active leads is required (that is, only one should be connected to the vaginal electrode). The ground pad is placed at the suprapubic site. During the 5-second alternating phases no stimulation is felt from the disconnected electrode. For greater stimulating effect, the vaginal electrode should have negative polarity. Current should be 80 to 100 PPS applied for 5 minutes in continuous mode, followed by 10 to 20 minutes in alternating mode (or surged mode, if available).

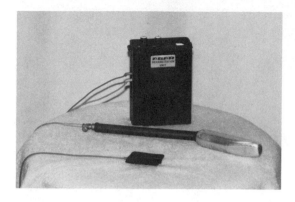

Fig. 5-4. Vaginal electrode connected to a lead from a compact EMS unit. The carbonized rubber electrode has been removed for this purpose. (Agar Corp.)

If interferential equipment is utilized for this purpose, a vaginal electrode should not be used. Instead, the four electrodes should be placed in a crossed pattern over the lower abdominal/pubic area so that the intersection of the two interferential circuits is just at the vaginal area. Tetanizing at 80 to 100 Hz for 5 minutes is suggested, followed by the sweep mode for 10 minutes.

If compact electrical muscle stimulation (EMS) (TENS-like) units are used, one of the carbon electrodes should be removed and the lead inserted into the vaginal electrode jack (Fig. 5-4). The secondary electrode should be placed in the suprapubic region, as with the others. A high rate (80 to 100 Hz) is suggested, with a medium pulse width (150 microsecs) and rapid rise rate for 20 minutes. (Since continuous stimulation with compact units requires manual key pressure by the patient, the tetanizing mode may be impractical.) Stimulation may begin immediately with the surged or interrupted mode at 4 to 6 second intervals.

If a vaginal electrode is not available for these procedures, the clinician may use an alternate technique. This often proves quite effective. With her hand, the patient holds a standard electrode over the perineum while lying supine with knees flexed.[6,10,11] The secondary electrode is placed suprapubic. The electrode from the patient's hand should be insulated with toweling or plastic to prevent current transmission via moist tissue contacts.

With all of the above, with stimulation a visible contraction of the perineal and adjacent musculature will be noted. The levator ani muscles as well as the perineal floor musculature are prime targets for this procedure. This should not be painful. *Patient tolerance takes precedence over visibility of contractions at all times with electrical stimulation.*

TRANSCUTANEOUS ELECTRIC NERVE STIMULATION

One form of electrical stimulation which is specifically designed to modify pain is transcutaneous electric nerve stimulation (TENS).[12-14] This noninvasive, simple and comfortable modality serves as a viable alternative to narcotic analgesia. Ideally, TENS should be utilized first rather than as a last resort, since heavy dependency upon narcotic medications will delay and minimize the effects of TENS administration. Once a diagnosis is made and the true cause of the pain known, TENS application should begin immediately to provide ongoing relief while further testing and procedures are undertaken. Too often, TENS is brought into the picture after drugs and other procedures have failed to relieve pain. Poor or minimal results may then follow with TENS. A trial period of at least 2 months is recommended in these instances, compared with 1 month for nonproblem cases.

The rationale for successful TENS is believed to be based upon one of the following two theories: (1) the Wall–Melzack[15] Theory of pain modulation via the gating mechanism in the substantial gelatinosa of the posterior horn; or (2) the concept of enhanced production of beta-endorphin, the endogenous pain-killer, by mild electric stimulation to the neural system.[5,14] In either case, most clinicians who have been utilizing TENS successfully for the past fifteen years agree on the benefits and advantages of this modality.

Several successful techniques with TENS involving various parameter selections and electrode placements have been reported by clinicians throughout the world. In most instances preferences are based upon prior successes. Each practitioner selects and administers TENS according to his or her training, experience, and comparative evaluations.

In my own 15 years with TENS, from early clinical investigation to standard procedures at our facility today, I recommend the following:

For acute pain, a high rate (80 to 100 Hz) with a medium pulse width (150 microsecs) and minimal intensities is recommended. Electrodes are placed at nerve roots, points of pain, and trigger and acupuncture points selected by the clinician. Treatment may be administered for one hour qid, or as needed. This technique tends to provide short term relief. (Some workers recommend longer treatment times, e.g., 2 to 4 hours. I have found the shorter periods effective while avoiding the undesired accommodation by the patient that is found with longer treatment times. The advent of modulated currents has helped to minimize accommodation; however, over the past 15 years my success with TENS has been based upon shorter but more frequent periods of stimulation.)

For chronic pain, a low rate (1 to 10 Hz) with a medium pulse width (150 to 200 microsecs) and minimal intensities is recommended. Electrodes are placed as with acute pain. Treatment may be administered for one hour bid, or *as needed*. This technique tends to provide delayed but longer-lasting relief, possibly due to increased levels of endorphin produced in the body as a result of the lower frequency. I do not suggest visible muscular contractions be elicited with TENS. (Some workers claim success with higher intensities.) Motor fibers are not the prime target with TENS; rather proprioceptive ("A") fibers are. (For specific electrode placements, I suggest consulting manufacturers' charts, current texts, and my own *Principles and Practice of Electrotherapy*[13,14] Fig. 5-5.)

TENS is a rapidly growing technique for labor and delivery. Used in many nations, with articles based upon successful utilization appearing more frequently,[16-26] this technique offers the patient and fetus drug-free deliveries.

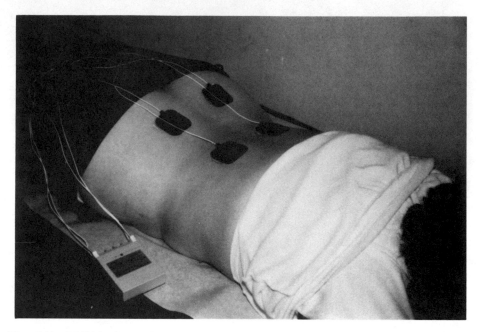

Fig. 5-5. TENS electrodes placed in a crossed pattern over the lower spine to influence the lumbosacral nerve roots. (Neurologix, Ltd.)

Apgar scores are reported to be good.[16-26] Israeli[17] and European reports[16,18,19] indicate good results in the form of reduced discomfort during and after deliveries, less dependence on narcotics throughout, no undesired side-effects, and mothers pleased with the procedure. The references cited here indicate a growing acceptance of this procedure by patients and obstetricians because of the noninvasive nature of TENS and the lack of dependency upon narcotics and other drugs during this particular period. Recent additions to the literature include material from sources in the United States, among which are the TENS manufacturers themselves, who are anxious to see TENS used more universally.[21-26]

Suggested protocols call for two separate circuits from a standard dual channel TENS unit. One pair of electrodes is placed at the mid-dorsal spine level and a second pair is placed at the distal spinal roots area of the sacral region. The proximal circuit is activated at the commencement of labor and the distal circuit is activated by the patient at each contraction. In the second stage of labor the distal electrodes are relocated anteriorly in a ''V'' pattern bilaterally at the suprapubic region. Parameter data, accurate electrode placements, and other details will be found in the references listed. Although not differing widely, the techniques reported with obstetric TENS suggest individual practitioners' preferences and successes. The physical therapist planning to use this modality should consult the references to ascertain common points of agreement before developing his or her own protocol[12-14,17,21,25,26] (Fig. 5-6).

Fig. 5-6. (A) Proximal electrodes extending from the bra strap line (T-8) downward to approximately L-1, bilaterally, about 3 inches apart. These electrodes are attached to one circuit from a dual channel TENS unit. The distal electrodes are placed bilaterally on both sides of the spine about 3 inches apart and as low on the body as possible without sitting on them. (*Figure continues*.).

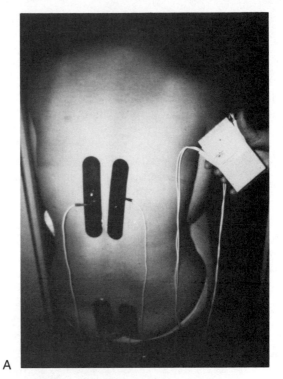

A

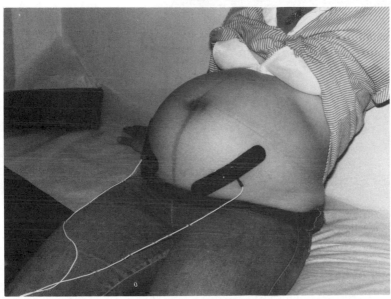

B

Fig. 5-6. (*Continued*). (B) At the 2nd stage of labor, the distal electrodes are transferred to the anterior abdomen. The recommended parameters are those for acute pain, i.e., high rate (80 to 120 Hz), medium pulse width (150 microsecs), and of sufficient intensity to block contraction pain without adding to it. The proximal circuit is turned on early on the day of delivery; the distal circuit is used during active labor. In some cases the proximal circuit is left on after delivery for additional comfort. (Fig. B from Kahn J: Principles and Practice of Electrotherapy. p. 147. Churchill Livingstone, New York, 1987.)

The effect of TENS on fetal monitoring equipment is controversial. Electronic filtration as installed by a bio-engineer and intermittent use of monitor may be recommended. The TENS can be turned off temporarily while the monitor is functioning; however, the technical points and methodology are best discussed with the bio-engineer at the facility involved.

As noted with many other electrotherapy procedures, additional assistance, e.g., exercises and prepared childbirth classes, is of extreme importance and should not be omitted.

Recent findings have indicated success using TENS to reduce morning sickness discomfort. This technique is an apparent spin-off from the success with postchemotherapy nausea using TENS. A high rate of 120 Hz with a medium pulse width of 150 microsecs, is advised, with minimal intensities. Electrodes are placed at the right acromial tip and at the traditional (right) "hoku" position (i.e. the web space between thumb and forefinger). It is recommended that treatment be administered for 30 minutes each morning. Interesting to note is that this technique does not seem to work if placed on the left (Fig. 5-7).

Studies are currently under way for the relief of dysmenorrhea and premenstrual pain using TENS. Electrodes should be placed at lumbo-sacral nerve roots and bilaterally in the suprapubic area. Parameter settings should be the same as for acute pain. viz, 1 hour, bid, or tid (Fig. 5-8). Although clinicians are optimistic about the effectiveness of TENS in these applications, no statistics or results are available as yet.

Sciatic radiculopathy, common during pregnancy and with gynecologic conditions, may respond well to TENS. Electrodes should be placed at the L5

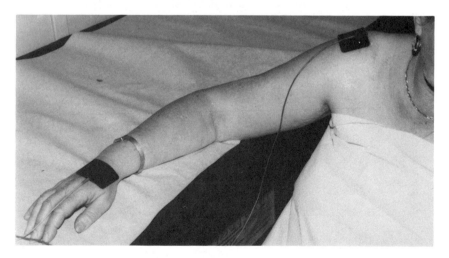

Fig. 5-7.   Electrodes placed at the right acromioclavicular joint and at the web space of the thumb/forefinger ("hoku") for morning sickness nausea. Rate: 80 to 120 Hz; width: 150 microsecs; minimal intensity: ½ hour each morning. (Kahn J: Principles and Practice of Electrotherapy. p. 148. Churchill Livingstone, New York, 1987.)

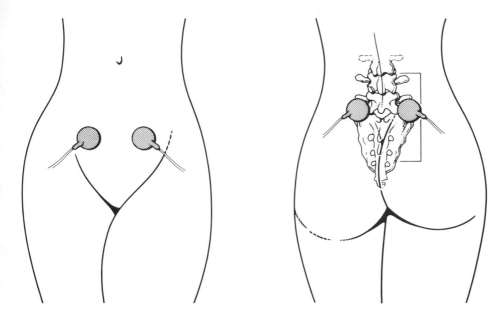

Fig. 5-8. For premenstrual pain, recommended electrode placements are at the lumbo-sacral nerve roots (L-4 to S-3) and suprapubic on the anterior abdomen. Rate: 80 to 120 Hz; width: 150 microsecs; minimal intensity: 1 hour several times daily.

nerve root, the midgluteus maximus acupuncture point, the popliteal acupuncture point, and behind the lateral malleolus, with parameters set for acute pain. These points are commonly used with low back pain and radiculopathies of the lower extremities. In most instances I prefer the intermittent technique of applying the therapy 1 hour several times daily rather than continuous or prolonged stimulation[12-14] (Fig. 5-9).

Most TENS models utilize biphasic or compensated monophasic wave forms, which are claimed to have no net direct current component. The positive phase, however, is usually of greater intensity and lends a slight positive bias to the current. This minimal polarity is not sufficient to favor ionic transfer to any great degree and so may be ignored. Rectangular pulses have been found to be more comfortable than the sharp, spiked wave forms, which generally are avoided by manufacturers because of patients reporting discomfort. (References to spike wave discomfort may be found in casual or informal reports throughout the literature.)

When a unit is used at home, the physical therapist should adjust all frequency and pulse width controls, modulation, etc., and have the patient set only the intensity. In this manner the continuity of stimulation may be reasonably controlled and the physical therapist may easily monitor any adjustments of the parameters which need to be made.

The previously mentioned techniques have been effective with all models and brands of TENS units used clinically. Although differing in wave form and

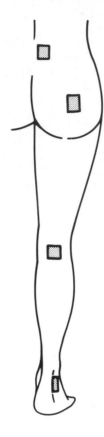

Fig. 5-9. The first, or "A," circuit of a dual channel TENS unit has electrodes placed at the L-5 nerve root on the affected side and at the center of the gluteus maximus. The second circuit has electrodes placed at the popliteal space and posterior to the lateral malleolus. Rate: 80-120 Hz; width 150 microsecs; minimal intensity; 1 hour, 3 to 4 times daily. (Kahn J: Principles and Practice of Electrotherapy. p. 139. Churchill Livingstone, New York, 1987.)

parameter limits, each of the many TENS units available today should produce satisfactory results in the hands of a trained and experienced clinician. I have not found any one to be superior to all others. With proper techniques, a skilled practitioner should be able to obtain favorable results with any of the current crop of TENS units. Conversely, poor technique on the part of the practitioner will lead to unfavorable results with even the best of units.

ULTRASOUND AND PHONOPHORESIS

Although I *have not* found ultrasound to be an effective modality for pain control, I *have* found phonophoresis an efficient analgesic; 0.5 percent to 1.0 percent hydrocortisone (anti-inflammatory), 5 percent lidocaine (anesthetic), 0.25 percent mecholyl (vasodilative), and 10 percent salicylate (decongestant) ointments offer the listed actions of the above molecules in a noninvasive procedure. When applied to associated nerve roots, this technique may offer a modicum of relief in certain instances involving radiculopathies and referred pain[27,28] (Fig. 5-10).

A particular problem during pregnancy is sciatic pain. Limited in several

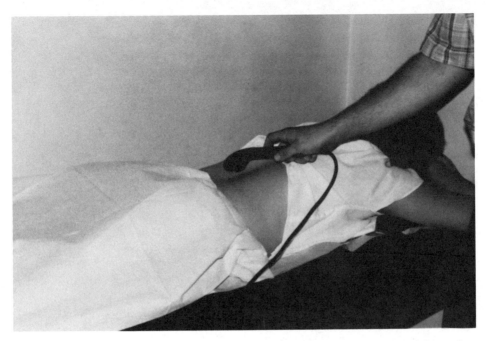

Fig. 5-10. Phonophoresis with 1.0 percent hydrocortisone ointment administered to the lower back and lumbosacral nerve roots. Usual US dosage is at 0.5-1.0 W/sq cm, continuous mode, for 3 to 4 minutes. (Mettler Corp.)

aspects of physical treatment during this period, the physical therapist must determine a safe yet effective procedure to relieve the painful symptoms of this neuropathic condition. Although effective, iontophoresis is questionable because the chemical is introduced into the patient. Likewise, phonophoresis may be contra-indicated because of the chemicals involved. Exercises designed specifically to reduce the tension along the sciatic distribution, i.e., those in which the patient's knees remain flexed, are certainly indicated. Superficial heating, e.g., infrared and gentle massage in the sidelying position, may be suggested. Also, TENS may be administered, although the long-term effects of TENS with pregnancy are still unknown. However, no untoward effects have been seen in the literature to date. I would not recommend the use of ultrasound on the lower back and sacral regions during pregnancy because of the interface heating characteristics of ultrasound, especially in the area of the sacral nerve roots, which are intimately involved with labor and delivery. Delicate placental tissues occupy the immediate vicinity as well. I have not used ice (cold packs) in my practice for this or other similar conditions with nonpregnant patients since I found early in my practice that blood pressures temporarily increase with the chilling effect. However, I favor other procedures, such as mild electric stimulation, TENS, or even the cold laser, leaving ice for the athletes and for patients with acute sprains or similar injuries.

As reported in the OB/GYN Newsletter (APTA),[26,29] utilization of ultrasound to alleviate the discomfort and congestion of the nipple during breast feeding has been found quite effective. One minute over the nipple/areola area at .5 to 1.0 W/sq cm apparently serves to "unclog" the impeded flow, with considerable relief. The mechanical characteristics of ultrasound are most likely the helpful agent here. (I have found no references to the use of ultrasound in cases of general mastitis.)

In an anatomical related condition, ultrasound has been reported to be of great value in the management of postsurgical sequela with breast augmentations (personal communication, Frank Herhan, M.D., Albuquerque, N.M., 1984). Often following silicone implantation, the implanted material coalesces into a hardened mass in the breast, necessitating a closed capsulotomy. This painful procedure consists of the surgeon compressing the hardened mass between his or her fingers until the mass bursts and is again reduced to a soft, pliable mass. Sources indicate that 3 to 4 minutes of ultrasound at 0.5-1.0 W/sq cm over the involved breast area will serve as a sclerolytic agent, softening the mass sufficiently to facilitate easy compression with considerably less discomfort for the patient. Daily massage of the affected area is mandatory to maintain the softened state. The proper massage technique can be taught to the patient by the attending physical therapist.

IONTOPHORESIS

The introduction of specific ions into tissues for therapeutic effect has provided substantial symptomatic relief when applied to nerve roots with gynecologic dermatomes. Vaginal iontophoresis with acetocholine was reported in the early literature[3]; however, this procedure has not been utilized in recent years since newer medications are available for the same physiologic purpose, i.e., vasodilation and increased local circulation. The clinician should remember that ionotophoresis is quite different from phonophoresis. In iontophoresis, ions are introduced electronically into the tissues whereas in phonophoresis, molecules are ultrasonically introduced. Ions and molecules differ widely chemically, physically, and in their physiologic effects. When scar tissue is involved, localized iontophoresis over the lower abdomen may be preferred to nerve root application. The physical therapist should suggest the appropriate ion and technique for each condition treated, based upon his or her specialized training in this area (Fig. 5-11). Specific techniques and protocols will not be covered in this chapter but may be found in manuals and handbooks designed specifically for this procedure.[12,13]

COLD LASER

The most recent advance in our field has involved the cold laser as a clinical modality.[30] A 1 mW helium/neon laser at 6328 AU has been shown to have favorable effects on localized pain, sclerolytic action on keloids and other scar tissues, as well as an apparent ability to penetrate cell walls to stimulate intracellular components, e.g., mitochondria responsible for metabolic changes

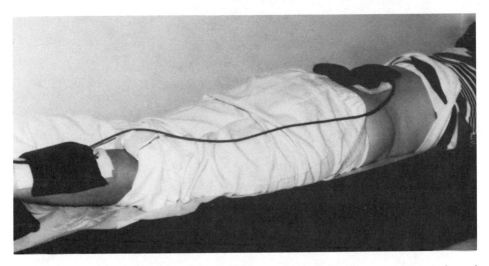

Fig. 5-11. Iontophoresis administered to the lumbosacral nerve roots. Note enlarged negative (indifferent) electrode on the distal calf. The particular ion introduced would be dependent upon the physiological effect desired. In this instance, it would be a positive ion. (Teca Corp.)

via DNA/RNA production.[31] Penetration is thought to be .8 mm directly and 10 to 12 mm indirectly with the refraction, reflection, dispersion, and absorption attending transmission of radiation through differential media.[33] At this writing, the full potential of the cold laser lies in the enhancement of healing open lesions.[33,34] This characteristic of the cold laser could be of great value in the management of gynecologic conditions, such as cervical erosions as well as minor surgical procedures. Current protocols call for only 90 sec/cm^2 wound surface of laser radiation at about 1 to 2 mm distance from the surface, 3 times/week to daily, if necessary. Results are usually obvious and noted after the first 3 to 4 treatments.

For applications with pain, the recommended techniques differ somewhat; applications should be applied from 15 to 30 seconds in direct contact with the patients' skin at known acupuncture points, trigger points, nerve roots, and pain sites. These points are identical with those used with TENS electrode placements (Fig. 5-12). (This should not come as a surprise since laser stimulation is acupuncture using a beam of light instead of a needle.) Treatment is administered daily, if indicated, as a procedure complete in itself or in preparation of other modalities.

OTHER MODALITIES

Important to mention at this point is that moist heat, massage, mobilization, hydrotherapy, and therapeutic exercise play important roles in the physical therapists' approach and should be included in all regimens where indicated and appropriate.

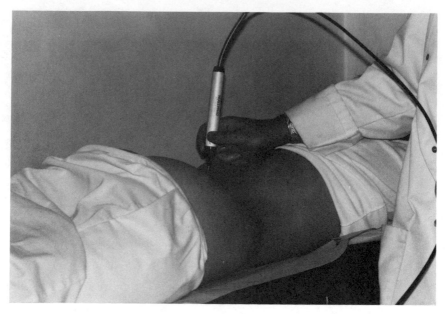

Fig. 5-12. The HeNe cold laser (6328 AU) administered to an acupuncture point for pain control. The recommended dosage is 15-30 sec with skin contact. (Dynatronics Laser Corp.)

SUMMARY

As an integral phase of physical therapy, electrotherapy should be included in the overall management of obstetric and gynecologic referrals, not as a panacea, but as a valuable adjunct to routine procedures. Our goal is to return the patient to normal health as soon as possible using any and all therapeutic means to accomplish this worthwhile objective. Electrotherapy is much too useful to be omitted from comprehensive planning. The licensed professional physiotherapist—or physical therapist, if you prefer—remains as the singularly best prepared practitioner in this discipline and should be included in the OB/GYN team whenever physical therapy is indicated.

REFERENCES

1. Jahier, Tillier: A case of amenorrhea treated with high frequency current. Jour de Radiologie et d'Electrol 28:55, 1947
2. Upton JR, Benson G: Results with local heating in PID. JAMA 121:38, 1943
3. Craig RL, Kraff H: Treatment of acute inflammatory masses of tubal origin by iontophoresis with acetyl-beta-methyl chloride. American Journal of Gynecology 45:96, 1943
4. Bengston BN: Sustained internal radiant heat in lesions of the pelvis. Archives of Physical Therapy 24:26, 1943

5. Sjoelund BH, Eriksson MBE: Endorphin and analgesia produced by peripheral conditioning stimulation. p. 587. In Bonica JJ (ed): Advances in Pain Research. Vol 3. Raven Press, New York, 1979

6. Vignes H: Electrotherapy of levator muscle of the anus during postpartum period and in some gynecologic conditions. Western Journal of Surgery 54:394, 1946

7. Malvern J, Edwards L: Electrical stimulation for incontinence. Medical Tribune, abstract, June 20, 1973

8. Moogaker AS: Management of stress incontinence in women. Geriatrics, June, 1976

9. Godec C, Cass A: Acute electrical stimulation for urinary incontinence. Urology 12:340, 1978

10. Rudinger EA: An electric device to strengthen pelvic muscles. The Female Patient, Nov 1979, reprinted in Ob/Gyn Newsletter, APTA 4:1

11. Hudgins AP: Electrical muscle stimulation in gynecology. Amer Prac 6:1695, 1955

12. Kahn J: Clinical Electrotherapy. 4th Ed. J. Kahn, Syosset, New York, 1985

13. Kahn J: Principles and Practice of Electrotherapy. Churchill Livingstone, New York, 1987

14. Manheimmer J, Lampe G: Clinical TENS. FA Davis, Philadelphia, 1984

15. Wall PP, Melzack R: Pain mechanisms, a new theory. Science 150:971, 1965

16. Augustinnson LE, Bohlin P, Bundsen P, et al: Pain relief during delivery by TENS. Pain 4:59, 1977

17. Tannenbaum J: Protocol for TENS in obstetrics. Hadassah Hospital, Jerusalem, 1980

18. Robson JE: TENS for pain relief in labour. Anesthesia 34:357, 1979

19. Bundsen P: Obstetrical anesthesia with TENS. Univ of Goteborg, Sweden, 1980

20. Tawfik MO, Badroui MH, El-ridi FS: The value of TENS during labor in Egyptian mothers. Cairo Univ., Egypt, 1980

21. TENS in Ob/Gyn Contributing authors Bulletin, Ob/Gyn Section, APTA, Vol 7 No 3, Sept 1983

22. TENS during labor and delivery: Boulder Memorial Hospital, Boulder, CO; reprinted Pain Control, No 39, Nov-Dec 1983, Staodynamics Corp., Longmont, CO

23. Keenen DL, Simonsen L, McCrann DJ: TENS for pain control during labor and delivery. JAPTA 65:1363, 1985

24. Grim LC: TENS for relief of parturition pain JAPTA 65:337, 1985

25. Ostman T, Wilszinsky C: Pain relief with TENS during labor and delivery. Unpublished article, April, 1985

26. APTA Bulletin 9:14, 1985

27. Nyborg WL, Ziskin MC: Biological Effects of Ultrasound. Churchill Livingstone, New York, 1985

28. Antich TJ: Phonophoresis. Journal of Orthopedics and Sports Physical Therapy 4:99, 1982

29. Shellshear M: Therapeutic ultrasound in post-partum breast engorgement. Australian Journal of Physical Therapy 27:1, 1981

30. Dynatronics Laser Corp., 270 West Crossroads Sq., Salt Lake City, Utah 84115

31. A Summary of Research in Biostimulation. Dynatronics Laser Corp., 270 W. Crossroads Sq., Salt Lake City, Utah 84115

32. Kleinkort J, Foley RA: Lasers. Clin Mngmt/APTA 2:30, 1982

33. Mester E: Effect of laser rays on wound healing. American Journal of Surgery Vol. 122, Oct 1971

34. Kahn J: Open wound management with the HeNe cold laser. Journal of Orthopedic and Sports Physical Therapy 6:203, 1984

6 | Relaxation Techniques in Prenatal Education

Yvette Woodrow

This chapter is an overview of relaxation theories and techniques as they apply to prenatal education and childbirth preparation. A review of the literature of the history of prepared childbirth training will be discussed, including a comparison of various childbirth preparation philosophies, general childbirth preparation techniques, and techniques for pain control. Additionally, different perspectives relative to the pain of childbirth, the physiologic bases for using relaxation techniques, alternative methods for relaxation, specific techniques, and the practicality of teaching these techniques to clients will be addressed.

Relaxation training is one component present in almost all prepared childbirth methods. The amount of emphasis placed upon it, however, varies considerably. A primary objective of these techniques is the reduction of pain during parturition. The focus of this chapter, therefore, will be on the purported effectiveness of relaxation techniques in coping with these sensations. Reference to other major components of prenatal education will be restricted to those relevant to the main theme.

PSYCHOLOGICAL AND PHYSICAL FACTORS IN INDIVIDUAL RESPONSES TO PAIN IN CHILDBIRTH

Several books on prepared childbirth suggest that labor is not really painful, or at least that it should not be painful unless there are complications.[1-4] According to these sources, psychological and physical preparation plus complete confidence in one's physician is all that is required in most cases to have a labor and delivery with only minimal discomfort. Because the pain of labor is worse than they had been led to expect, many parturient women are left feeling inadequate, and this sense of failure is often compounded by the "attitude of an indoctrinated husband."[5]

Pain in labor exists if it is so perceived by the woman experiencing it. Determinants in the perception of pain include the intensity and duration of the stimulus (of which a wide variety occur in labor experiences), and the pain threshold (which differs among individuals and which may fluctuate within the same person).[5]

Psychological and Physiologic Variables

Shelia Kitzinger states, "Pain is never merely a sensation."[6] It has both a physical and psychological aspect. Yet, while the process of childbirth is considered a physiologic function, it differs from other physiologic functions in that it occurs only a few times in a woman's life. The mechanical distention of childbirth is unparalleled by any other process.[7] Any resultant tissue damage is reported by pain receptors.[8] Dr. Lee Buxton explains that physical stimuli arising during labor are transmitted via several receptors to the cortex. During contractions there is mechanical pressure on nerve endings and blood vessels in the uterine muscles, as well as pressure on the pelvic floor and the birth canal by the fetal presenting part. Stretching of the cervix, uterine ligaments, peritoneal covering of the uterus, and the perineum also occurs. These areas contain numerous pain receptors.[9]

Buxton proposes that pain occurring at the time of uterine contraction may well be caused by ischemia of the uterine wall, particularly during the transition phase between the first and second stages of labor when the contraction period often lasts longer than the rest period between contractions.

On the psychological side, the mental state of a person can modify the incoming painful stimulus so that its perception is either increased or decreased.[8] This mental state is influenced by preconditioning, traditional practices, and psychosocial factors such as anxiety about the upcoming process and results, the woman's attitude to the coming child, the woman's feelings toward her body, and the kind of relationship she has with the child's father.[6] Many of the current obstetrical practices often administered routinely, such as intravenous fluids (IVs), fetal monitoring, and vaginal examinations, may add to maternal anxiety. All of these factors can influence the threshold and determine the amount of pain a woman is prepared to accept.[5] Since the mind and body are inseparable, for techniques to be effective consideration must be given to both aspects.[10]

Is There Pain During Labor?

Once it has been recognized that some pain does occur, the pain of labor for the woman experiencing it can either have a negative or positive connotation. An immense qualitative difference exists between pain which is experienced as a result of a task which achieves a goal and pain which is part of a destructive process such as disease or injury.[6] Maplestone commented, "With so many variables capable of producing an almost indefinite number of combinations, there is no such thing as a standard labor."[5] It is essential for all people involved with the expectant mother or couple to bear these facts in mind and not set unattainable goals of behavior for the mother. The mother must be allowed to view herself and her personal labor experience as unique and not have to meet expectations imposed by others.[11]

Many childbirth educators do not speak about the pain of parturition. They feel that even the mention of pain may be enough to induce its presence in labor.[5,8] This kind of attitude leaves many women totally unprepared for what they may encounter. Yet, some of the difficulty in acknowledging pain during childbirth stems from inadequate evaluation of pain in quantitative terms owing to the lack of instruments with which to objectively measure the sensation of pain.[7] Statistics on the percentages of pain experienced and scales of measurement vary from one source to another. One article describes only 5 percent of first labors as being painless.[12] The most common figure for painless labor is between 7 and 14 percent.[7] Another article describes as high as 25 percent of deliveries as being painless (this figure included multiparas). Overall, the following generalization may be made: Approximately 25 percent of childbirths are mildly painful; 25 percent are moderately painful; 25 to 40 percent are extremely painful; and 10 to 15 percent have been described as intolerable. In spite of being general and nonspecific, these figures point out that a very large percentage of women do experience moderate to severe pain and thus should be at least forewarned during prenatal instruction.

PHYSIOLOGIC BASIS FOR RELAXATION TRAINING

There are measurable physiologic changes which have been recorded consistently in association with varied physical states. These include the fight or flight response, the relaxation response, the fear–tension–pain syndrome, Pavlovian conditioning, and gate control theory.

Fight or Flight Response

The fight or flight response[13,14] is the body's mechanism to prepare itself for confrontation or escape, and is initiated when a person is faced with a situation which requires adjustment of behavior, such as in response to pain, fear, or apprehension. The fight or flight response is believed to be controlled by the hypothalmus. The activation of the sympathetic nervous system results in the secretion of specific hormones: adrenalin or epinephrine and norepinephrine or noradrenalin. These hormones increase heart rate and blood flow to the muscles and elevate blood pressure, metabolism, and breathing rate. If unresolved, as when neither fight or flight is the proper course of action, these changes result in increased levels of tension in specific muscle groups and translate into the following posture: shoulders elevated, elbows and hands flexed and jaw clenched. Continual elicitation of this response to meet stresses of daily living, without discharge of energy, may lead to habitually increased levels of tension and possibly to heart attack and stroke.[14]

The Relaxation Response

The relaxation response, as described by Dr. Herbert Benson, is the antithesis of the fight or flight response.[14] He believes both responses are controlled by the hypothalmus. Therefore, evoking the relaxation response will counteract the harmful cumulative effects of the fight or flight response. Initiation of the relaxation response occurs through concentration on a passive state. Physiologic changes which have been observed to accompany this state include decreases in oxygen consumption (significantly lower than in sleep), blood lactate (purported to be associated with anxiety), metabolic rate; heart rate, and blood pressure (in subjects with prior elevation of blood pressure). An increase in alpha wave intensity and frequency has also been noted.[14] Benson associates the relaxation response with "an altered state of consciousness." He considers it an altered state "simply because we do not commonly experience it and because it usually does not occur spontaneously; it must be consciously and purposefully evoked."[14] This response, then, should be the goal of relaxation training for labor and delivery.

Fear–Tension–Pain Syndrome

The fear–tension–pain syndrome was first described by Dr. Grantly Dick–Read, a British obstetrician. His theory is that women have the preconceived idea that labor and delivery are painful processes. This notion, he believes, is culturally instilled and encourages fear. This fear signals the fight or flight response when uterine contraction occurs. Along with the effects previously noted in relation to the fight or flight response, Read contends that the sympathetic nerve supply to the uterus supplies the circular fibers of the cervix and lower uterus, and thus their excitation inhibits dilatation. As the longitudinal fibers continue to contract, two muscle groups, then, are working in opposition, resulting in excessive tension and leading to "real pain." Thus Read postulates that "through the misinterpretation of noninjurious stimuli, a painless natural function is made into an extremely painful and abnormal condition"[1] (Fig. 6-1).

Read's method of preparation, therefore, is to provide accurate information about the childbirth process and have the patient practice physical relaxation and thus disrupt the vicious cycle. He believes that "if the body is completely relaxed it is impossible to entertain the emotion of fear."[1] The main criticism of Read's theory is that he views fear in a limited way, believing that

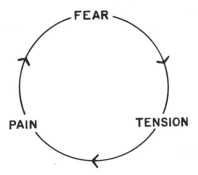

Fig. 6-1.   Read's fear–tension–pain cycle.

it is exclusively culturally produced. He does not allow for the physical pain-producing components of birthing. Many also believe Read's method contains a large number of suggestive techniques, although Read does not concur with this sentiment.[7]

Pavlovian Conditioning

Buxton reviewed a complex Russian interpretation of the psychoprophylactic method based on Pavlovian conditioning.[9] A simplification is that the neurophysiologic mechanism of pain transmission is interrupted by a conditioned reflex produced through frequent practice and the remolding of women's conscious expectations of labor. The sensations from labor are thus to be blocked or sublimated by the clinician or labor support person providing a counterstimulus at the right time. In this approach, emphasis is placed on the "importance of the function of the cerebral cortex as the higher center of pain perception."[9]

Gate Control Theory

The gate control theory of pain control was presented by Melzak and Wall in 1965 and may shed some light on how operant conditioning can decrease pain awareness.[10,15,16] Briefly, the main components involved in this theory are the following:

1. Small diameter "C" fibers. These fibers are slow firing, lasting many seconds, and are believed to carry pain impulses. They are distributed throughout the spinal cord but lie predominantly in the anterior portion outside the dorsal column. They have access to the hypothalamus, thalamic nuclei, and the limbic system in the forebrain and thus have some connection with the affective–motivational aspects of pain.

2. Large diameter "A" fibers. These fibers are rapid firing (200 ms) and carry mechanical stimulation such as touch, rubbing, joint movement, and

vibration. They ascend in the dorsal column to reach the thalamus. These provide the "spaciotemporal discriminative capacity for pain."[16]

3. Central control mechanism. "The central control mechanism . . . influences the gate control system through efferent fibers descending to spinal levels and entering the substantia gelatinosa, where they join in the modulation of sensory input."[15] Thus, psychological functions can modify, at the spinal level, the sensations perceived.

The interaction of these three components leads to the pain gate mechanism. Perception of pain depends upon the balance between "C" and "A" fiber inputs and the modification of these inputs by the central control mechanism. Simply, a decrease in "A" fiber stimulation with an increase in "C" fiber stimulation opens the gate, creating excessive sensitivity to pain. Massage, touch relaxation, and operant conditioning techniques are believed to increase "A" fiber input, which closes the gate and decreases pain perception.[15] Modification by the central control mechanism (psychic component), which can be accessed through specific training techniques, can additionally close the gate.[15] Examples of techniques which can influence the central control mechanism in a gate closing manner are attention focusing, cognitive rehearsal, autosuggestion, and emotive imagery work. Although this theory is being modified as more is learned about neurophysiology, it lends some credence to Chertok's view, expressed in 1959, that analgesia can be produced psychosomatically by "blocking," or through a central modification of pain perception through the intervention of affective factors.[7] This description is in keeping with the gate control theory.

REVIEW OF THE LITERATURE: EFFECTS OF GENERAL CHILDBIRTH PREPARATION

In 1980 Rosemary Cogan presented a fairly comprehensive review of past studies on the effects of childbirth preparation.[17] What follows is an overview of her work.

Studies of Childbirth Preparation Classes

In studies that controlled for differences between women who elected and those who did not elect to attend childbirth preparation classes, positive benefits were clearly and reliably demonstrated for the prepared group. A common criticism of these studies has been that they were biased by self-selection or that the population in these classes did not reflect an accurate sample. Cogan, however, reviewed other studies, which included control groups electing childbirth preparation but not receiving classes either because of inaccessability or because classes were full.[18] These control groups had birth experiences similar to subjects who did not elect to attend or who did not receive classes. Therefore, Cogan concluded that childbirth preparation itself had a positive effect on the birth experience."[17]

Benefits of Childbirth Preparation

Benefits of childbirth preparation include the following:

Analgesia and anesthesia. Consistent evidence is available that less medication is required during labor and delivery for gravidas who receive childbirth education.[17,19,20]

Pain during labor. Most studies indicate that childbirth preparation has helped to reduce pain during labor and delivery.[8,17-20]

Fetal state during delivery. Childbirth preparation has been associated with more stable fetal heart rate and lower incidence of fetal distress during labor in a few studies.[17]

Attitudes of women. Most studies conclude that childbirth preparation leads to a greater awareness by the mother at birth and to a more positive attitude toward childbirth.[17]

Less frequent use of forceps. Six studies examined by Cogan reported less frequent use of forceps in the prepared groups.[17]

Stress/anxiety reduction. From research in situations other than childbirth, several authors have concluded that information presentation preceding distressing experiences can reduce the emotional impact of stress.[8,18,21] Beck and Siegel state that "there is experimental evidence to indicate that anxiety (or fear) can be reduced by a variety of treatment paradigms. Anxiety reduction procedures with empirically demonstrated effectiveness include systematic desensitization, modeling, flooding, reinforced practice and various cognitive strategies."[21]

PSYCHOANALGESIC METHODS OF PAIN CONTROL USED IN CHILDBIRTH CLASSES

The research reviewed tends to examine the effects of childbirth preparation as a whole. Childbirth preparation courses, however, consist of multiple components. Thus, the isolation of those specific factors responsible for the therapeutic results produced is virtually impossible.[21] Only Jacobson used his "progressive relaxation" method exclusively in preparing his patients for labor and delivery. He based his conclusions on case reports between 1930 and 1954 and did not utilize principles now considered essential in research design. He believed that pregnant women could be trained more efficiently using strictly physiologic methods, which is what he considered his "progressive relaxation" method to be. In regard to the literature available on psychological strategies used to deal with pain in general, many of the studies either focused on the effectiveness of childbirth preparation techniques with experimentally induced pain, or compared results with childbirth relaxation techniques.

Stevens categorized five major psychological strategies found in laboratory studies to effectively reduce pain perception.[8] They include systematic relaxation, cognitive control, cognitive rehearsal, the Hawthorne Effect, and systematic desensitization.

Systematic Relaxation (Tense–Relax)

Systematic relaxation involves contracting to varying degrees a muscle group for a set length of time and then releasing it to gain relaxation of that particular muscle group. In this manner, several muscle groups are tensed and relaxed often in a set pattern working from distal to proximal muscle groups. Systematic relaxation has been found effective in increasing pain tolerance in a number of studies. (For more information on progressive relaxation and tense–relax, see the section, Specific Techniques, below.)

Cognitive Control

Cognitive control is a strategy in which the subject concentrates on other mental activities rather than on the incoming pain sensation. There are two variations of cognitive control used in childbirth preparation: dissociation technique and interference technique.

Dissociation Technique

Stevens describes dissociation technique as "concentrating one's attention upon a nonpainful characteristic of the stimulus."[8] Concentrating on labor contractions as muscular contractions of the uterus rather than as labor pains is such a technique. This strategy has been found successful in increasing both endurance and pain threshold.

Interference Technique

Interference technique can be broken down into two components, distraction and attention focusing.

Distraction. Distraction "involves a passive perceptual interference" using an exterior stimulus, e.g., listening to music or a story. Several studies have shown this technique to be effective in increasing endurance to painful stimuli, especially the slow-onset type.[8]

Attention Focusing. Attention focusing involves an active, intentional and purposeful mental activity which focuses on another process, either mental or physical, e.g., concentrating one's vision and mind upon a specific object. Stevens and Heide found this technique more effective in reducing pain perception and increasing pain tolerance when combined with feedback relaxation strategies.[20]

Cognitive Rehearsal

Cognitive rehearsal requires providing the subject with a clear explanation of what will be involved in the forthcoming experience. A number of studies have found this strategy effective in the reduction of pain perception.[8,21] One of these studies, according to Stevens, concluded that for cognitive rehearsal to be more effective, both subjective and objective information had to be clearly and accurately given and the subjective information had to be verified by the subject's own experience.[8]

The Hawthorne Effect

The term Hawthorne effect is used to denote the special attention given the subject by the experimenter which may affect the outcome. Beck and Siegel feel that many studies are invalid because they do not include an attention-placebo treatment group to negate this effect.[21] Stevens contends that the Hawthorne effect has interesting implications for prenatal education. The childbirth educator and the coach have the role of experimenter in providing the special attention for the expectant mother. This, in itself, may affect the success of the techniques used for pain management.[8]

Systematic Desensitization

Formally a part of clinical psychiatry, this procedure "combines systematic relaxation, cognitive rehearsal, cognitive dissociation and the Hawthorne effect for the treatment of specific fears and anxieties."[8] Stevens contends that childbirth preparation methods are an informal form of systematic desensitization for "childbirth fear of labor pain." One study, according to Stevens, found both prepared childbirth classes and systematic desensitization effective in decreasing childbirth anxiety in women exhibiting high anxiety; however, the latter approach was significantly more successful. Stevens concluded that women with high anxiety need more intense childbirth preparation.

Beck and Siegel commented on the same study, reporting that the "systematic desensitization group . . . had significantly shorter labours . . . and were rated by the obstetricians as experiencing less pain and manifesting less restlessness."[21]

A study by Bobey and Davidson used four groups: control, relaxation, anxiety, and cognitive rehearsal. Heat and pressure pain stimulators were used. Results indicated that the relaxation group was more effective in dealing with both types of pain.[23]

Beck and Siegel also critically reviewed prepared childbirth studies, including those mentioned above. Shortcomings were found in all studies; however, they drew the following conclusions:

> There is substantial evidence to indicate that the temporal combination of the imagination of feared events with relaxation leads to substantial reductions in the self-report, behavioral, and psychophysical manifestations of anxiety.

> Preliminary findings indicate that a combination of certain cognitive restructuring techniques with relaxation might produce a tolerance to pain which rivals the effects of morphine.

> Much of the research on anxiety reduction suggests that treatment procedures such as relaxation training and exposure to anxiety-related stimuli are most effective when delivered within the context of a well organized and carefully planned treatment program.[21]

The implications for prenatal educators are many. Scientific evaluation of specific techniques should be explored, and the least effective techniques discarded. Classes need to be planned with consideration given to strategies based on research in order to provide the most beneficial program to prospective parents.

EVOLUTION OF PREPARED CHILDBIRTH

In the 1920s, a few members of the medical community began to show interest in the psychological aspects of labor and delivery.[24] One of the British physicians was Dr. Grantly Dick–Read, who in 1933 published his book, *Childbirth Without Fear,* postulating his fear–tension–pain syndrome. This book is still a common reference for prenatal education. His ideas were used and adapted to other methods of childbirth preparation. Figure 6-2 diagrams the evolution of childbirth preparation stemming from Dick–Read.

The interest in preparation for childbirth continues, spurred on by the feminist movement. Many women want to take an active part in the delivery of their children.[25] Also many women tend to be highly motivated to do whatever they believe will benefit the health of their children prior to parturition. Prenatal education, therefore, could also be considered a "preventive program" in the health care field, and as such, hopefully, will continue to evolve.

POPULAR PSYCHOSOMATIC METHODS USED IN
CHILDBIRTH PREPARATION

Chertok and Buxton extensively reviewed the varieties of psychosomatic methods applied to childbirth preparation.[7,9] They concluded that almost all contained some type of learned relaxation, patterned breathing, and informa-

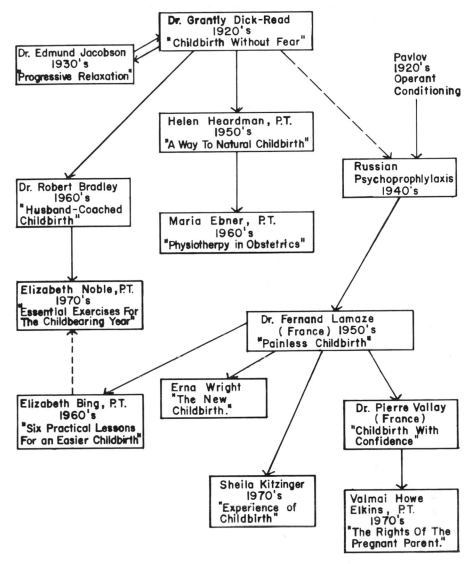

Fig. 6-2. Evolution of prepared childbirth.

tion about labor and delivery. The only exception was the previously mentioned program of childbirth preparation by Jacobson. Although each procedure had a somewhat different emphasis, individual techniques overlapped and were variations of a similar theme; in each, some form of psychophysical device was taught to help women cope with the sensations of labor. Figure 6-3 illustrates some of these similarities and differences, especially in regard to relaxation and breathing techniques.

	Personality Or Method	Origin Or Basis	Relaxation Technique						Breathing				Exercises	Husband/Coach	Information
			Tense-Relax	Auto-Suggestion	Differential Disassociation	Massage	Touch-Relax	Imagery	Level I Diaphragmatic	Level II	Level III	Level IV Panting			
NATURAL CHILDBIRTH	Dick-Read Method	Based on Dr. Grantly Dick-Read's Fear-Tension-Pain Cycle.	■	▨					■			■	■	■	■
NATURAL CHILDBIRTH	Bradley Method	Started by Dr. Robert Bradley's Stress on Husband-Coaching. Influence by Dick-Read.	■		▨	■		■	■ [a]				■	■	■
NATURAL CHILDBIRTH	Elizabeth Noble R.P.T.	Emphasizes Prevention & Control through Physical Preparation.	▨ [b]			■	■		■				■	■	■
PSYCHOPROPHYLAXIS	Lamaze Method	Patterned after Russian Psychoprophylaxis. C Incorporates Pavlovian Conditioning. Uses Directive Psychological Analgesia to Modify the Perception of pain.	▨			■	■		■	■	■	■	■	■	■
PSYCHOPROPHYLAXIS	Elizabeth Bing R.P.T.	Lamaze Derivitive	▨		▨	▨			■	■	■	■	■	■	■
PSYCHOPROPHYLAXIS	Valmai Howe Elkins Australian P.T. Working in Canada	Lamaze Derivitive Patterned after Dr. Pierre Vallay Who Worked With Dr. Lamaze.	■	■	■	■	■	■	■	■	■	■	■	■	■ [d]
PSYCHOPROPHYLAXIS	Shelia Kitzinger British Child-Birth Ed. Psychosexual Method. e	Lamaze Derivitive Promotes Harmony In Mind & Body.	■	■		■	■	■	▨	▨	▨	▨	■	■	■
OTHER	Autogenic Training (Used Extensively By Prill in Germany)	Combines a Psychological and Exercise Approach As a Technique For Subconscious Control of Thought Processes.				■							■		■
OTHER	Edmund Jacobson M.D. Progressive Relaxation	Practiced to Obtain Complete Subconscious Neuro-Muscular Control.	■												

Fig. 6-3. Subjective analysis of similarities and differences of some current popular childbirth preparation methods. ■ Strong emphasis; ▨ moderate emphasis; □ slight emphasis, no emphasis, or unknown emphasis. (This figure is a subjective analysis based on several references. [1,2,22,26–29] Also used as references were lecture notes from presentations by Valmai Howe Elkins, Sheila Kitzinger, and a Bradley Teacher Certification Workshop.) (*a*) In the Bradley method, diaphragmatic breathing is preferred as the most relaxing and physiologically advantageous form of respiration. (*b*) Elizabeth Noble advocates the Mitchell method of physiologic relaxation, to be described later in this chapter. (*c*) The term psychoprophylaxis has become synonomous with the Lamaze method, although there may still exist some differences with

ALTERNATIVE METHODS

Several other techniques have been infrequently used during labor and delivery and are related in some fashion to relaxation. These techniques will be reviewed briefly.

Hypnosis

According to Dr. Herbert Benson, hypnosis is defined as "an altered state of consciousness which is artificially induced and characterized by increased receptiveness to suggestions."[14] He has not recognized a consistent specific physiologic state which occurs as a result of hypnotic trance; however, when deep relaxation is the hypnotic state suggested, the relaxation response has been evoked.[14] Women may choose to go through parturition in a hypnotic trance or may choose posthypnotic suggestion. Either method is capable of producing an anesthetic effect.[2]

Hypnosis is not utilized more frequently because the process is very time consuming and because not everyone is capable of being hypnotized. In Walker's estimation, only 5 percent of the population can achieve a deep trance, 35 percent a medium trance, and only a light trance can be achieved by the balance.[2]

According to Chertok's investigation of psychosomatic methods in childbirth, there is little quantitative difference between the production of an experimental analgesia created by hypnotic means and that created by other psychological means. Only a difference of degree could be documented.[7] Chertok noted that in certain individuals relaxation could induce hypnoid states in which those individuals were very receptive to suggestion. Chertok also cited an article by Mandy and coworkers which reported that "hypnosis and relaxation are phenomena which are in a reciprocal relationship. Hypnosis is a continuum which runs from simple relaxation right up to somnambulism. The method of induction of a light trance is almost the same as that of the technique of relaxation."[7] On the other hand, Read and Jacobson, among others, felt very strongly that relaxation had nothing to do with this hypnoid state.

Biofeedback

In biofeedback, the subject learns voluntary control over automatically regulated body functions, such as muscle tension, heart rate, blood pressure, and temperature. Training sessions in which specific equipment gives immedi-

---

the Russian application. (*d*) Valmai Howe Elkins puts very strong emphasis on patients' rights within the Health Care System. (*e*) Parfitt comments on Kitzinger's psychosexual method as offering a sexual/sensual awareness to birthing and its preparation: "Birth is the climax of a sexual process and the mother has most success when she can open up, relax and feel trusting."[26]

ate feedback on the state of whichever physiologic variable is being monitored are employed.[30,31] Some techniques of relaxation, such as tense/relax, autogenic, imagery, or a combination of these, as well as passive concentration on the change in a specified direction, may be used during the training sessions.

Biofeedback to learn relaxation for labor and delivery is a relatively new area. Only a few studies have been reported but preliminary results seem promising.[31] The tremendous advantage in biofeedback is that the subject receives immediate feedback as to how well she is controlling her functions. Controlled changes are often obtained within a few sessions. Disadvantages to this method are that costly equipment is required, and the equipment is often not available for home use.

John Paul Brady reports that in studies where biofeedback and relaxation training have been compared, they were equally effective. He therefore concludes that relaxation training is the more convenient of the two methods.[30] If available, however, the use of biofeedback to reinforce training in those subjects who have difficulty learning to relax or who do not feel they are obtaining results would be invaluable. According to Brown, a most important aspect of biofeedback is that "it shifts the focus of control of the self from external to internal dependence."[31] The subject no longer relies on external devices or others; "the control of his physiologic functioning can and does come from within; and he learns that he can depend on his internal control systems."[31]

Yoga

Yoga classes are offered prenatally. This technique combines physical and breathing exercises, concentration, meditation, and relaxation techniques. According to Stella Weller, the yoga student learns to use the breath as a powerful tool against tension. Yogic theory contends that "smooth regular breathing has a calming influence on the mind; shallow irregular respiration contributes to anxiety and restlessness."[32] The concentration directs attention to one activity and maintains this focus for a period of time. Yogic relaxation techniques consist of local and systematic application. Meditation and the yogic philosophy are important aspects of this program. Walker comments, "Yoga is practiced for purposes of centering–finding the truth within and the meaning of life."[2] One principle behind this method is that "one learns to control circumstances to some extent, rather than be totally at their mercy."[32]

Transcendental Meditation

Transcendental meditation (TM) involves a fairly simple technique. The subject is given a secret word, sound, or phrase, called a mantra. This is to be mentally perceived. The meditator silently repeats the mantra over and over again while sitting in a comfortable position. During each session, the assumption of a passive attitude and the disregard for other thoughts is important to the recitation of the mantra. This practice should be observed twice daily for 20 minutes.[14]

The relaxation response previously shown to be elicited by TM has also been noted in hypnosis (when the suggested state is deep relaxation), in yoga, in autogenic training, and to some extent in progressive relaxation. Benson believes the elicitation of the relaxation response incorporates four basic elements: a quiet environment, a mental device, a passive attitude (one should not be concerned about how well he or she is doing), and a comfortable position. An aspect of the relaxation response measured by Benson in some techniques is that of increased alpha wave sensitivity. In his book *The Pain Game*, Norman Shealy describes the following rates of "rhythmic electrical activity" in the brain[10]:

Beta State: 14–22 pulses/second; wide awake awareness when the mind is conscious of what is outside it.

Alpha State: 8–13 cycles/second; occurs during close, intent concentration when the mind is not so susceptible to distraction.

Theta State: 4–7 cycles/second; mind becomes even more withdrawn from what is happening externally as in deep hypnosis.

Delta State: 1–3 cycles/second; sleep occurs

Shealy theorizes that if a person can purposefully reach the level of the "alpha or theta states and remain there, he can suppress his pain."[10] Essential to reaching this state is "total concentration on a single thing or on nothing at all."[10] Relaxation techniques as well as the other methods discussed above fulfill these criteria. Thus, it seems valid to conclude that these techniques are all different means to attain the same end. The practiced application of whatever method chosen should enable the individual to attain this "altered state" or, as Chertok states, the "state of relaxation which is beneficial and curative."[7]

RELAXATION TRAINING AND RELATED TECHNIQUES
Prospective

"All supplementary relaxation techniques focus upon awareness of internal states, i.e., attention is directed inwardly instead of the usual outwardly directed attention. This change in the normal person's perspective entails a learning process, and the aids supplied by autosuggested phrases, comparing relaxation with tensing, and sitting quietly becoming aware of the self, act as self-teaching devices to explore personal territory that has been so long screened from awareness."[31]

Objectives of Relaxation Training in Prenatal Education

The following is a list of relaxation training objectives:

1. To help conserve energy. Relaxation of voluntary muscles during the first stage of labor will save the mother's strength for the exertion necessary for active participation in delivery.
2. To reduce mental stress/anxiety. Authors frequently state that relaxation and anxiety are mutually exclusive.[23,31] A relaxed person cannot be anxious, nor when anxious can be truly relaxed.
3. To help control or ride over the pain of labor. The studies previously cited indicate that relaxation techniques can increase the pain threshold and endurance to pain; reduced perception to pain has also been postulated.
4. To facilitate labor and delivery. A well-known theory states that cervical dilatation occurs more easily when the woman can remain in the relaxed state.[1,9]
5. To serve as a coping skill for life. Relaxation skills once mastered are not forgotten; although aimed specifically at labor and delivery, they can and should be incorporated into everyday living to deal with stressful situations.[13,28]

Specific Techniques

Internal Locus of Control (self-directed)

Neuromuscular Techniques

(a) Tense–relax. Tense–relax is the most common type of relaxation taught in prenatal classes. Tense–relax is a derivative of the Jacobson method of "progressive relaxation," although Jacobson's method was much more specific and required a fairly extensive training period.[33] This technique involves tensing a set of muscles, noting the tension, and then releasing the tension while remaining aware of the sensations. This sequence is repeated in a progressive fashion with different muscle groups in turn. The instructor might proceed, for example, from lower extremities to upper extremities to trunk and to face, followed by total body relaxation. The relaxation sequence might be repeated a second time with reduced tension and then a third time with no tension. Throughout the process the patient should concentrate on relaxing each area in turn.[34]

(b) Physiological Relaxation (Mitchell method). Physiological relaxation, as introduced by Laura Mitchell, is based on contraction of muscle groups which are antagonists to those groups contracted in positions of stress. Joint position sense and skin sensation are used to help retrain the subject to recognize the relaxed position thus obtained. A definite sequence of contractions is used to achieve this. The sequence consists of three definite instructions which the subject gives to herself for each area: (1) Do the chosen movement; (2) Stop doing it; (3) Register the new position of the joint concerned and skin sensation (if applicable). These three components are used

in a systemathic method throughout all the regions of the body, resulting in a body awareness of the ease position for general relaxation.[13]

(c) Selective Tension (Disassociation). In selective tension exercise, one area of the body is tensed while the subject attempts to keep all other areas relaxed. This technique is supposed to simulate the contraction of the uterus during labor. The coach is often incorporated in this conditioning type of exercise by giving the orders, checking for tension, and giving feedback on relaxation. A frequent criticism of this method as a preparation for labor is that uterine contractions are not under one's control, as are the tensions produced during the exercise, and therefore the conditioning may not be considered valid by the woman in labor.[13]

(d) Breathing Techniques. Breathing techniques are restricted in this discussion to those used as a complement to relaxation. One exercise involves mentally saying the word "calm" on inspiration and saying "relaxed" on expiration, since natural relaxation occurs with expiration; "The rhythm of slow deep breathing assists relaxation."[28] Another exercise uses the image of tension flowing out or being stripped away with expiration. Although one observes the body's natural rhythm in breathing patterns, no overt attempt is made to control it.

Mental Techniques

(a) Imagery. In imagery, concentration on a mental image rather than on the physical state is used to produce the relaxation response. This technique, as well as all the others, requires daily practice to develop effectiveness; also, each individual must decide which images are the most suitable for personal use. Teaching this method in a group setting such as prenatal classes presents some difficulties in this regard; however, a handout with numerous suggestions may aid people to choose for themselves what image is right for them. Individual counseling is ideal.

(b) Emotive Imagery. Emotive imagery involves having the subject picture herself first in a tension-producing situation, then in a relaxing one; e.g., the subject may first imagine herself getting into a cold lake for a brisk swim, then stretching out and relaxing on a sunny, warm beach.[29]

From this point, Kitzinger suggests moving on to imagining situations involving emotional conflict, such as when walking alone on a dark street. Recognition of the muscular tensions involved is followed by deliberate, complete relaxation. With practice, the aim is to be able to imagine the same tension-producing situation and meet it with relaxation. This concept was also part of Jacobson's progressive relaxation method.[33]

(c) Color and Numbers. Some people find the mental visualization of colors or numbers easier to associate with relaxation. Dr. Frederick Lenz describes a method of inducing relaxation by color association. First, different parts of the body are consciously relaxed while the subject thinks of a specific color. After adequate practice, the subject should be able to relax those areas just by thinking of the color alone.[35]

Various methods of relaxing using numbers are also advocated. One technique involves counting backwards from 100; the subject relaxes more with each number. Another technique involves visualizing the number 3 while exhaling and mentally repeating the phrase, "complete body relaxation." The next step is to visualize the number 2 while exhaling and mentally repeating the phrase, "complete brain and nervous system relaxation." The number 1 is visualized in a similar fashion and the mental phrase is "oneness, mind–body harmony."[31] This technique may work well as a trigger for the relaxation response after one has learned neuromuscular relaxation via another method.

(d) Attention Focusing. Some find using a visual focal point for concentration useful. When used in the Lamaze method, this technique is usually associated with more intricate breathing patterns. Focal point concentration can be useful for those individuals who are uncomfortable relaxing with their eyes closed. Prior conditioning can be utilized by practicing relaxation while looking at a familiar object which, if small enough, can be brought into the labour room.

Other individuals are able to obtain muscular relaxation and release from tension through listening to music or poetry. This auditory attention focusing could also be utilized to condition suitable subjects to cope effectively with labor.

Mental focusing occurs whenever any of the techniques described above are faithfully practiced and when one or two aspects of a technique are emphasized. Even the techniques listed under "external locus of control" can become a focus of attention if the woman can internalize the stimulus provided by the coach. This can only be achieved through frequent practice.

(e) Autosuggestion. Dr. Lee Buxton states, "The essence of autosuggestion is to develop by constant practice a wish, aim or desire of the conscious mind . . . by means of communication with what is considered to be the subconscious mind."[9] The subconscious is presumed to have "considerable control over visceral function."[9] Suggestions to the subconscious are made by mental or vocal repetition of the desired change when the subconscious is considered to be most active, such as just before sleep or in a quiet introverted mood. This mood may be connected with increased alpha wave production. Overt efforts of will by the conscious mind, therefore, cannot be effective in producing desired changes, as it is the subconscious which is influenced while the subject is in a passive state.[9] Well controlled relaxation provides such an environment. Numerous authors use different terms to describe the same state, i.e., "restful alertness,"[28] "deep stages of relaxation,"[31] "state of neuromuscular release,"[29] trance,"[1] "deep relaxation,"[13] "alpha and theta states,"[10] state of relaxation which is beneficial and curative,"[7] and "state of controlled relaxation."[36]

Some of the authors discussed above combine autosuggestion with their own procedures. Kitzinger suggests, "If the woman nearing full term uses this time [when practicing relaxation] to think about being in labor and to visualize the physiological processes which she has learned occur during the first and second stages of labor, and to look forward to the experience whilst in this state of neuromuscular release, she will also be allowing herself the additional aid derived from controlled autosuggestion."[29] Application of cognitive rehearsal is also employed here. Autosuggestion is not generally utilized in prenatal preparation at present; however, application of this method combined with relaxation may lead to the psychoanalgesia women seek.

Combined Neuromuscular and Mental Techniques

Autogenic Training (AT). Although many of the above techniques are to some extent combinations of physical and mental methods, nowhere are they as well combined as in AT. This technique was developed by Dr. H. H. Shultz, a German neurologist. The goal of AT is for the subject to attain deep relaxation by himself. Six exercises, carried out sequentially, concentrate on bodily sensations. These sensations include heaviness in the limbs, warmth in the limbs, regular cardiac and respiratory rhythms, a feeling of warmth in the abdomen, and a coolness in the forehead.[7,9,10,14,31] Shealy describes AT as a form of "sensory biofeedback."[10]

All of the above methods have one thing in common—concentration is focused on a specific item, be it physical tension, a relaxed feeling, image, sound, or sensation. This concentration does not involve monitoring how well one is doing. A causal detached attitude is very important. As Noble states, "It is very important to release the mind and body; as long as you continue to speculate and evaluate how you are getting along, participation is blocked."[28]

External Locus of Control (coach-directed)

Touch Relaxation. This method, associated with Sheila Kitzinger, has recently become a popular technique taught in prenatal classes. The aim of this technique is to develop a "nonverbal communication based on touch" between the pregnant woman and her labor coach.[29] In this type of conditioning exercise, the coach learns to recognize areas of tension and the woman learns to respond to his touch through frequent practice. Some women who have difficulty visualizing images often find this method more helpful.

Massage. In some prenatal classes the coaches are taught a basic, rudimentary massage to help relax their partners. Massage of areas prone to tension and sites of perceived pain in labor is demonstrated.

Coaching Techniques. Various techniques aimed at supplementing relaxation during labor are taught to the coaches. These include timing contractions, helping maintain a regular breathing rate, reinforcing the partner's relaxation techniques by verbalizing images, giving the orders for relaxation, utilizing touch relaxation, and being encouraging. These coach-oriented exercises should be included in all childbirth preparation programs which are given for couples, or where a woman will be accompanied into labor by a parent or friend.

PRACTICAL APPLICATION

There are a wide range of methods for relaxation training. What suits one person will not necessarily suit another. Therefore, an attempt should be made to find the right method for each person. This may mean that relaxation itself is not a suitable technique for some. Allowing for individuality, then, is not an easy task considering the present design of prenatal classes, which range from 4 to 40 couples per class. Perhaps some time has to be allowed for individual counseling.

All relaxation techniques require frequent practice to be effective. A novice should practice a minimum of 20 minutes a day, and twice daily is preferable, to master the techniques and to be able to achieve deep relaxation in the few months available to her before labor commences. In a survey in 1962, Buxton reported, "It was almost the unanimous opinion of physiotherapists and preparators that a sizeable percentage of the women taking prepared childbirth courses did not follow through with the instruction exercises which they were supposed to pursue at home."[9] The same can still be said today.

Perhaps a more feasible way to teach relaxation would be to offer supplemental classes in this area for those desirous of learning this art and willing to put forth the effort necessary. The simpler techniques, as well as the coach-oriented methods, could be introduced in the regular classes while leaving the more complex techniques for those interested in additional instruction.

A concensus exists among those involved with autogenic training and progressive relaxation techniques that these methods appear "to be more specifically adaptable psychologically to certain types of women with appropriate intellectual capacity and background."[9] Other qualities called for are perseverance and the capacity for concentration. Internal locus of control is essential.

Another aspect to consider is the individual's psychological orientation. A person who relaxes by running 2 miles is not as likely to feel comfortable in the passive state of relaxation. A more active way of coping with labor needs to be taught to these people. Perhaps more complex breathing patterns are much more likely to appeal to and work for this personality type.

PROPOSALS FOR APPLICATION

Considering the above points, the following proposal for more effective presentation of relaxation techniques in childbirth education is suggested. Some way must be found to assess the individual's suitability for these different aspects of the program. A questionnaire may be one way to discover some of these characteristics of the learner (entry behavior). Participants could then be given information, both verbally and written, during regular classes on two different specialized approaches: relaxation and breathing techniques. The decision relative to the pursuit of more intensive supplemental training in either technique should then be left up to them. Admission to these two programs should be placed on a contract basis, i.e., the instructors agree to impart their specialized skills and give directions wherever needed while the participants agree to follow through with the required daily practice. To be effective, these classes should be small so that individuality can be stressed.

Preparation for childbirth, carried out as directed above, may form a more solid basis from which to analyze results of the use of the different components now offered in prenatal education.

SUMMARY

The different perspectives on pain suggest that the expectation of painless labor and delivery is unrealistic. Childbirth preparation classes must prepare women for unique individual experiences. Therefore, a delicate balance of the amount of emphasis given to this topic must be achieved. This balance is not easily accomplished in a group setting.

The relaxation response as described by Benson is of considerable importance as it establishes physiologic manifestations which can be objectively measured. Review of the literature on childbirth education indicates positive effects for laboring women. Studies involved specifically with relaxation techniques suggest positive results with experimental pain, but their application to parturition needs further investigation and analysis of the various components.

The evolution of childbirth preparation programs, their similarities and differences, and the use of alternative methods have greatly influenced the development of relaxation techniques. All methods, however, incorporate four basic elements: a quiet environment, a mental device, a passive attitude, and a comfortable position. The relaxation response seems to be the desired goal.

Specific relaxation techniques vary within prepared childbirth classes, but a combination of muscular relaxation, cognitive rehearsal, and autosuggestion may be essential for consistent psychoanalgesia. However, more effective preparation and more valid research may be facilitated through a different, more individual approach to relaxation. An adaptation of Glaser's basic teaching model may help the reader develop this individualized style (Fig. 6-4). Educators should remember that the principles of teaching need to be applied when planning prenatal programs.

CONCLUSION

The essential skill of learning to relax in our high-pressured society can no longer be disputed. Physical therapists can make a valuable contribution in this area of preventive medicine. As Brown so aptly states, "The goal is the voluntary control of the tension-relaxation dimension of muscles and the inexpressible but subjectively known awareness that gives one the ability for control."[33] "Most powerful is he who has himself in his own power."

ACKNOWLEDGMENTS

The author would like to thank Dave Woodrow for the illustrations and Dorothy Boran and Linda O'Connor for their editorial assistance with this work.

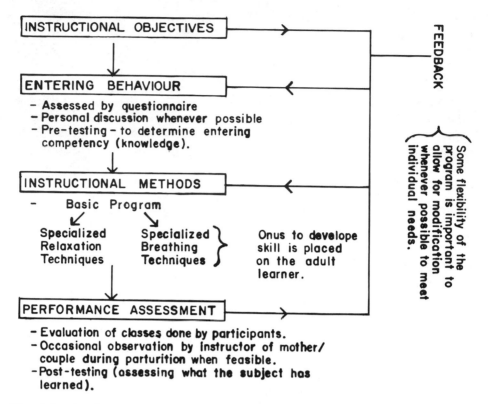

Fig. 6-4. Application of Glaser's basic teaching model to childbirth preparation classes.

REFERENCES

1. Dick-Read G: Childbirth Without Fear, the Principles and Practice of Natural Childbirth. Harper and Brothers, New York, 1944
2. Walker M, Yoffe B, Gray PH: The Complete Book of Birth, from Grantly Dick-Read to Leboyer, a Guide for Expectant Parents to all Methods of Birth. Simon & Schuster, New York, 1979
3. Fenlon A, McPherson E, Dorchak L: Getting Ready for Childbirth, A Guide for Expectant Parents. Prentice-Hall, Englewood Cliffs, New Jersey, 1979
4. Hungerford MJ: Childbirth Education. Charles C Thomas Publisher, Springfield, Illinois, 1972
5. Maplestone PA: Pain relief in labour. Med J Aust 2:610, 1977
6. Kitzinger S: Pain in childbirth. J Med Ethics 4:119, 1978
7. Chertok L: Psychosomatic Methods in Painless Childbirth, History, Theory, and Practice. Translated from the 2nd French edition. Pergamon Press, New York, 1959
8. Stevens RJ: Psychological strategies for management of pain in prepared childbirth I: A review of the research. Birth and the Family Journal 3:4:157, 1976
9. Buxton CL: A Study of Psychophysical Methods for Relief of Childbirth Pain. WB Saunders, Philadelphia, 1962

10. Shealy CN: The Pain Game. Celestial Arts, Millbrae, California, 1976
11. Clark AL: Leadership Techniques in Expectant Parent Education. 2nd Ed, Springer-Verlag, New York, 1973
12. Lennane J, Lennane J: Hard Labour, A Realist's Guide to Having a Baby. Victor Gollane, London, 1977
13. Mitchell L: Simple Relaxation, The Physiological Method for Easing Tension. John Murray, London, 1977
14. Benson H: The Relaxation Response. William Morrow, New York, 1975
15. Downey JA, Darling RC: Physiological Basis of Rehabilitative Medicine. WB Saunders, Philadelphia, 1971
16. Werner JK: Neuroscience, A Clinical Perspective. WB Saunders, Philadelphia, 1980
17. Cogan R: Effects of childbirth preparation. Clin Obstet Gynecol 23:1, 1980
18. Cogan R, Henneborn WJ, Klopper F: Predictors of pain during prepared childbirth. J Psychosom Res 20:523, 1976
19. Cogan R, Henneborn WJ: The effects of husband participation on reported pain and probability of medication during labour and delivery. J Psychosom Res 19:215, 1975
20. Stevens RJ, Heide F: Analgesic characteristics of prepared childbirth techniques: Attention focusing and systematic relaxation. J Psychosom Res 21:451, 1977
21. Beck N, Siegel L: Preparation for childbirth and contemporary research on pain, anxiety, and stress reduction: A review and critique. Psychosom Med 42(4):429, 1980
22. Jacobson E: Relaxation methods in labour. Am J Obstet Gynecol 67:1035, 1954
23. Bobey MJ, Davidson PO: Psychological factors affecting pain tolerance. J Psychosom Res 14:371, 1970
24. Hirshberg M: The history and philosophy of childbirth education. Physiotherapy Canada 27(2):83, 1975
25. Doering SG, Entwisle DR, Quinlan D: Modeling the quality of women's birth experience. J Health Soc Behav 21:12, 1980
26. Parfitt RR: The Birth Primer, A Source Book of Traditional and Alternative Methods in Labour and Delivery. Running Press, Philadelphia, 1977
27. Bradley RA: Husband-Coached Childbirth. Harper & Row, New York, 1965
28. Noble E: Essential Exercises for the Childbearing Year, A Guide to Health and Comfort Before Your Baby is Born. 2nd. Ed. Houghton-Mifflin, Boston, 1982
29. Kitzinger S: The Experience of Childbirth. 4th Ed. Pelican Books, Middlesex, England, 1978
30. Brady JP: Behavioural medicine: Scope and promise of an emerging field. Biol Psychiatry 16(4):319, 1981
31. Brown BB: Stress and the Art of Biofeedback. Bantam Books, New York, 1977
32. Weller S: Preparing for childbirth the yoga way. Australian Nurses Journal 10:11, 1981
33. Jacobson E: Progressive Relaxation, A Physiological and Clinical Investigation of Muscular States and Their Significance in Psychology and Medical Practice. 4th Impression. University of Chicago Press, Chicago, 1946
34. Cautela JR, Groden J: Relaxation, a Comprehensive Manual for Adults, Children and Children with Special Needs. Research Press, Champaign, Illinois, 1978
35. Lenz FP: Total Relaxation, the Complete Program for Overcoming Stress, Tension, Worry and Fatigue. Bobbs-Merrill, Indianapolis, 1980
36. Heardman H: A Way to Natural Childbirth, A Manual for Physiotherapists and

Parents-to-be. E and S Livingstone, Edinburgh, 1952 --Physiotherapy in Obstetrics and Gynaecology, Including Education for Childbirth. E and S Livingstone, Edinburgh, 1951

SUGGESTED READINGS

Ebner M: Physiotherapy in Obstetics, Including Education for Childbirth and Postnatal Restoration. 3rd Ed. E and S Livingstone, Edinburgh, 1967

Macfarlane A: The Psychology of Childbirth. Harvard University Press, Boston, 1977

Astbury J: The crisis of childbirth: Can information and childbirth education help? J Psychosom Res 24:9, 1980

Frazier LM: Using biofeedback to aid relaxation during childbirth. Birth and the Family Journal 1(4):15, 1974

French DJ, Leeb CS, Boener GL: Theoretical applications of biofeedback hand temperature training to prepared (lamaze) childbirth training. Percept Mot Skills 37:326, 1973

Herman E: The use of transcutaneous nerve stimulation in the management of chronic pain. Physiotherapy Canada 29(2):65, 1977

Marshall K: Pain relief in labour, The role of the physiotherapist. Physiotherapy - Journal of the Chartered Society of Physiotherapy 67(1):8, 1981

Mulcahy RA, Janz N: Effectiveness of raising pain perception threshold in males and females using a psychoprophylactic childbirth technique during induced pain. Nurs Res 22(5):423, 1973

Scott JR, Rose NB: Effect of psychoprophylaxis (lamaze preparation) on labour and delivery in primiparas. N Engl J Med 294(22):1205, 1976

Stone CI, Demchik-Stone DA, Horan JJ: Coping with pain: A component analysis of lamaze and cognitive-behavioural procedures. Psychosom Res 21:451, 1977

Wallach HS: Psychological and physiological childbirth related variables affecting pain in labour. Newsletter 64 - Obstetrical Division, Canadian Physiotherapy Association. Winter 1982-83

Zho D, Dighe J, Basmajian JV: EMG biofeedback and chinese chi kung: Relaxation effects in patients with low back pain. Physiotherapy Canada 35(1):13, 1983

Zimmerman-Tansella C, Dolcetta G, Azzini V, et al: Preparation courses for childbirth in primiparas. A comparison. J Psychosom Res 23:227, 1979

7 | Physiologic Adaptations and Considerations of Exercise During Pregnancy

Edwin Dale
Karen M. Mullinax

In the past, pregnancy has been considered by many physicians and their patients as a time of pampering and confinement of the mother and her fetus. In fact, obstetricians during the first half of the twentieth century calculated an estimated date of confinement (EDC) as the date for predicting delivery of the child. However, with the increased awareness of and participation in various types of physical fitness and exercise programs, especially jogging, many women during the past 10 years have expressed dissatisfaction with confinement and have essentially stated their wish to continue, or even begin, exercise programs during their pregnancies. Confronted with this revolution, obstetric health care providers have been faced with many questions, e.g., What are the effects of exercise on the mother? the fetus? What types of exercises can be carried out? How much? What are the legal and ethical issues of exercise prescription? And, finally, Is exercise during pregnancy safe, necessary, or desirable in improving the quality of labor and delivery or the outcome of pregnancy?

Interestingly, the historic perspective provides some basis for and many thoughts relating to maternal fitness and pregnancy outcome. The following examples illustrate this point. In Biblical times, Hebrew slave women had easier (more rapid) labor than their less physically active Egyptian mistresses—"They are lively, and are delivered ere the midwife came to them." Aristotle in the third century B.C. attributed difficult childbirth to a sedentary life-style. In more modern times the pendulum has swung in both directions. Eighteenth century philosophy encouraged exercise, albeit with strong limitations. In 1892, Stacpoole wrote, "When you neglect, risk or injure your own health during pregnancy, you do a direct injustice to, and commit a real crime against your baby."[1] This statement obviously suggests a more moderate approach to work and exercise during pregnancy. The nineteenth century also brought forth the first scientific attempts at examining the relationship of maternal activity and pregnancy outcome. These studies continue into the present time.

At the beginning of the twentieth century, the themes of moderation in exercise and the need for fresh clean air were the dominant recommendations despite the absence of any scientific proof for either. The amount of exercise which the prospective mother should take could not be stated precisely but what was definitely said was that she should stop the moment she began to feel bad. Further, "Walking is the best kind of exercise. . . . Most women who are pregnant find that a two to three mile walk daily is all they enjoy and few are inclined to indulge in six miles, which is generally considered the upper limit."[1] Additional restrictions included prohibitions against horseback riding, tennis, and, interestingly, excessive walking. Throughout the 1930s there were attempts to promote increased physical activity for pregnant women. The major contributions of this period were Vaughn's prenatal exercises, emphasizing squats as a method of strengthening the perineal musculature, Read's progressive specific breathing patterns, and Lamaze's psychoprophylactic method of childbirth which appeared during this decade.

Exercise advice from 1940 to 1960 differed little from the conservative 1920s; all of the previous admonitions were maintained and emphases given to moderation and regular walking in the open air. A more complete account of this portion of the historic perspective is found in a recent book.[1]

Within the past two decades, however, more and more women began participating in many different sports activities and physical fitness programs and at all levels of fitness and competition. The views of earlier years were considered old-fashioned and outmoded and were rejected by many. Today, many women want to know if they can continue their sports activity during pregnancy, and others ask if an exercise program will enhance or improve their pregnancy outcome or shorten labor and delivery. Much of today's exercise emphasis is on aerobic dancing, cycling, and running as part of essential health maintenance.[2,3] The proportion of American women who exercise during their pregnancies is difficult to determine. In a recent publication it was estimated that some 85 million citizens are involved in fitness programs and 25 million jog regularly.[4] Women of reproductive age constitute a significant portion of the active American public. In 1982, the *Mortality–Morbidity Weekly Report* (MMWR) reported that a survey of California women aged 18 to 34 showed only 10.8 percent admitted to a sedentary lifestyle.[5] Also, many women work outside the home during their pregnancies. In the period 1970 to 1973, 42 percent of all pregnant women were reported to be in the work force. In view of the current trend toward increased physical fitness, we must be aware of where our patients are coming from and where they want to go in terms of expediting their pregnancies, labors, and deliveries.

Maternity care providers are often confronted with issues of safety and maternal/fetal effects of exercise during pregnancy as they attempt to counsel their pregnant patients on the advisability of exercise. The literature available on exercise during pregnancy is varied. Much is anecdotal and appears in popular magazines.[6-8] Women read about Olympic gold medalists competing in the first trimester of their pregnancy or of women competing in races of 10 km or participating in marathons in the latter half of their pregnancies. Health care providers also read these success stories of exceptional athletes in their own professional journals.[9] Much of the early research on exercise during pregnancy was done on the exceptional athlete.[10-13] The question is, What about the everyday athlete who is pregnant? What specific information does one give her concerning the advisability of beginning or continuing her exercise program during pregnancy?

In attempting to answer these questions we shall examine in the following sections some of the physiologic adaptations during pregnancy, the impact of exercise occurring simultaneously, the animal model, and human clinical studies. We shall also examine some concerns about the performance of exercise during pregnancy and conclude with a review of current recommendations.

PHYSIOLOGIC RESPONSE TO EXERCISE DURING PREGNANCY

Exercise imposes additional requirements on the respiratory, cardiovascular, musculoskeletal, and metabolic systems beyond those changes already established because of pregnancy. As pregnancy is a state of intimate interaction between mother and fetus—interaction which may be disturbed by physiologic stresses that would be inconsequential to a nongravid woman—several aspects of exercise cause concern for possible effects on the fetus.

Cardiovascular Changes

The circulation of a pregnant woman may be characterized as hyperdynamic. The heart rate is increased, the pulse is rapid and bounding, and there is increased blood flow to several organ systems and the rapidly enlarging uterus. Total blood volume increases by 35 percent or more during pregnancy and cardiac output is elevated in pregnant women. Cardiac output increases approximately one third above resting nonpregnant levels. The major portion of the increase occurs by 8 to 10 weeks after the last menstrual period.[14]

Maintenance of the elevated stroke volume and increased cardiac output is dependent on adequate venous return. Venous pooling from prolonged standing or occlusion of the vena cava by the gravid uterus when assuming the supine position can decrease stroke volume and cardiac output. These phenomena are seen in pregnant laboratory animals which do not assume an upright posture.[15]

Exercise elicits a greater increase in cardiac output in the pregnant woman. This occurs not only because she is moving a greater body weight; the cardiac output increase for a standard amount of exercise is greater during pregnancy than in the nonpregnant state. In response to moderate exercise, the corresponding increase in cardiac output is progressively smaller as pregnancy nears term. This progressive decline in cardiac reserve can also be attributed to obstruction of the vena cava secondary to the enlarging uterus, which contributes to peripheral pooling of blood.[16]

In a study conducted at Emory University on cardiovascular changes during the second and third trimesters, Wilder, Campbell, Law, and Gianinio[17] evaluated resting heart rate (HR) and blood pressure (BP) measurements in groups of exercising and nonexercising women. The findings of their study failed to demonstrate a difference in these parameters between pregnant women who participated in a 4 week group active exercise program and those pregnant women who did not exercise. Their findings further indicated that there were no significant changes in HR and BP from the beginning to the conclusion of the exercise program; their studies thus fail to support previous research suggesting pregnant women are trainable through a regular active exercise program.[18] Small sample size (4 experimental and 7 control), nonrandom selection and assignment, and limited matching for gestational age were cited by the authors as weaknesses of this study.

Pulmonary Changes

During pregnancy the respiratory center in the medulla becomes further sensitized to carbon dioxide. The change is effected by increased circulation of progesterone during pregnancy. The result is a lowering of carbon dioxide tension in maternal blood by approximately 25 percent. The sensation of breathlessness with mild exercise which is frequently reported by pregnant women is probably a manifestation of increased sensitivity to carbon dioxide. Other respiratory changes which impact upon pregnancy include a rise in minute volume which at term is about 40 percent above nonpregnant levels. The increase in minute volume is brought about by an increase in tidal volume and not by increase in respiratory rate. Minute ventilation during exercise also increases during the latter months of pregnancy. The rate of increase remains proportional to the work load on a bicycle ergometer. These alterations indicate that during pregnancy, metabolic efficiency of the body remains the same, but energy cost of a given work load is increased. As a result of increase in body weight during pregnancy, more oxygen is required to exercise during pregnancy. Therefore, a woman reaches maximal exercise capacity at a lower level of work during pregnancy than in the nonpregnant state.[14]

The increase in minute ventilation results in the normal hyperventilation state of pregnancy with a decline in arterial PCO_2 levels to approximately 30 mm Hg and a rise in arterial PO_2 of approximately 105 mm Hg.[1]

The alterations in cardiopulmonary functioning produced by pregnancy have been studied in relation to exercise. Guzman and Caplan[19] found no difference in the physiologic response to exercise in pregnancy. However, they found that the pregnant woman reached her maximum work capacity at a lower level of work than in the nonpregnant state.

Knuttgen and Emerson[20] also studied 13 pregnant women and found that exercise did not constitute a severe physiologic stress during pregnancy when weight bearing, lifting, or walking was not involved. Where body weight impacts on the cost of exercise, as in treadmill walking, the increased cost during pregnancy is proportional to the increase in body weight. Similar cardiorespiratory responses were also noted in a study by Artal et al.[21]

Musculoskeletal Changes

Alterations in the musculoskeletal system may also affect a pregnant woman's performance. Estrogen and the ovarian hormone relaxin produced by the corpus luteum induce softening of connective tissue ligaments and joints, predisposing them to stress and strain. The resulting relaxation of the fibrous ligaments and cartilage is particularly apparent in increased motility of the pelvic joints, which can be painful and impact on the ability to perform exercise. In the last trimester of pregnancy, there is decreased mobility in the wrist and ankle joints despite the increased relaxation of the ligaments. These changes are felt to be a result of water retention in the connective tissue of the joints. This presents with ankle, pedal and pretibial edema and sometimes paraesthesias in the hands as carpal tunnel syndrome.[1]

The enlarging uterus also accentuates lumbar lordosis, which affects balance and center of gravity. Those exercises which require rapid movement and coordination may predispose the pregnant woman to a fall.

Approximately 30 percent of all pregnant women experience weakening of the central fibrous tissue seam between the rectus abdominus muscles of the abdomen. This can result in a separation called diastasis recti. Abdominal strengthening exercises need to be modified to prevent further separation if the diastasis is larger (greater than 3 finger breaths). (More detailed information and management techniques for diastasis recti and other musculoskeletal disorders can be found in Chapters 2, 3, and 4.)

Endocrine Changes

The placenta can be viewed as the major endocrine organ of pregnancy. Its production of human placental lactogen (hPL), human chorionic gonadotrophin (hCG), estrogen, and progesterone have a major impact on pregnancy.

A key role is played by hCG in maintaining the corpus luteum of pregnancy; hCG reaches a peak between 8 to 10 weeks of gestational age. It is postulated that hCG has a role in fetal development, e.g., induction of fetal testosterone secretion from the fetal testis or certain regulatory functions of the fetal adrenal.

The activities of hPL include increased insulin production, increased peripheral resistance to insulin, lypolysis, and nitrogen retention. This activity leads to a "diabetic effect" in pregnancy. Altered carbohydrate metabolism also can contribute to metabolic ketoacidosis and hypoglycemic episodes in pregnant women whose intake of calories has not been sufficient. Exercise has an impact on these calories which should be increased in active pregnant women to prevent ketoacidosis and other manifestations of diabetes mellitus.

The primary action of the placental steroids estrogen and progesterone is to enhance growth of the reproductive organs—the uterus and breasts. Estrogens also increase the elastic properties of the uterine muscle and encourage contractility of the muscle while progesterone works to keep the uterine musculature quiet and nonactive. Estrogens influence the growth of the ductal system of the breasts while progesterone influences the glandular portion of the breasts. Fat content and vascularity also increase in the pregnant breast secondary to the stimulation of the two hormones.

Progesterone encourages generalized smooth muscle relaxation throughout the pregnant body. This contributes to a slower gastrointestinal tract, causing constipation, and to venous dilation, causing varicosities in pregnancy. Progesterone also resets the respiratory center and encourages sensitivity to PCO_2 blood levels. This results in the "hyperventilation" of pregnancy and the sense of breathlessness many patients have even at rest. Progesterone additionally resets the thermoregulatory center, raising the temperature 0.5 percent F over usual readings. Both of these changes impact greatly on exercise tolerance.

Other endocrine changes include an elevated prolactin level from the pituitary, which assists in breast milk production. The actions of corticotrophin (ACTH) and thyrotropin (TSH) do not appear to change during pregnancy. Follicle stimulating hormone (FSH) and luteinizing hormone (LH) decline to luteal phase levels, leading to an anovulatory state during pregnancy.

Thyroid function tests are affected by estrogen. Thyroxin-binding globulin (TBG) elevates total T_3 and T_4 during pregnancy. Symptoms of a hyperactive thyroid are common during pregnancy and include a bounding tachycardia and intolerance to heat. The thyroid is not overactive during pregnancy.

The adrenal glands produce increased concentrations of steroids during pregnancy. Circulating catecholamines, norepinephrine, and epinephrine do not change during pregnancy until labor and delivery. Increases in epinephrine and norepinephrine levels have also been noted in response to moderate treadmill exercise in pregnant women. Increase in norepinephrine was greater in these cases and is of potential concern because of its ability to stimulate uterine activity and perhaps induce preterm labor.[22]

Cortisol plasma levels are also elevated in the first trimester and continue to rise until delivery. Plasma concentration reaches levels encountered in Cushing's syndrome, although there are no clinical signs. It is felt that clinical signs are not present because of the competitive actions of other circulating hormones, especially progesterone.

The two mineral corticoids of the adrenal cortex, aldosterone and lldeo-xycorticosterone (DOC), are also elevated during pregnancy. Aldosterone production is regulated by various system changes—renin angiotensin, which reacts to alterations in mean arterial pressure, sodium and potassium levels, and by direct stimulation of ACTH. Increased circulating estrogens stimulate liver production of angiotensinogen, the substrate for renin to form angiolencin II. Angiotensin II stimulates the production of aldosterone. Decreased mean arterial pressure in pregnancy triggers the release of renin. Renin encourages sodium retention and fluid expansion to raise arterial pressure. Theoretically, these changes should encourage hypertension. Hypertension does not result, however, because of the counteractive effect of progesterone, which prevents sodium retention and excessive potassium loss. The hypertensive actions of angiotensin II are counteracted by estrogen. The net effect is normal blood pressure, but with normal accumulations of fluids seen as dependent edema in ankles, feet, and pretibial areas of the pregnant woman.

These pronounced endocrine effects can impact on the exercise tolerance levels of a pregnant woman and should be given consideration when prescribing an exercise program.

NUTRITIONAL NEEDS FOR ACTIVE PREGNANT WOMEN

The nutritional needs of active pregnant women have not been studied extensively. Based on general nutritional recommendations for pregnant women, some guidelines can be made for those women involved in athletic activities.

Caloric/Energy Requirements

An additional 300 calories per day have been recommended for all pregnant women in order to compensate for the increased basal metabolic needs during pregnancy. This energy requirement will rise as activity increases and/or as pregnancy progresses. Energy requirements in late pregnancy, when the woman must move a larger body weight, are probably more than 300 calories per day.

The energy needs of an active pregnant woman will vary based on the exercise performed (i.e., running at 36 weeks of pregnancy will require more caloric intake to maintain appropriate weight gain than riding a stationary bicycle at 13 weeks of pregnancy). Additional calories to maintain an adequate total weight gain of 25 to 35 pounds will be required. Artal recommends 500 calories per day for women who are maintaining a 30 minute daily exercise program during pregnancy (vs 300 calories per day for sedentary pregnant women).[1] If the rate of gain per visit or total weight gain of pregnancy does not appear to be adequate, additional calories may be needed. A diet high in complex carbohydrates is advised during pregnancy in order to prevent ketonuria and replenish muscle glycogen loss as a consequence of exercise.

Protein Requirements

The usual dietary intake of protein in the United States exceeds the recommendation for pregnancy and is probably adequate for active pregnant women. Artal recommends a diet providing 12 percent of the energy consumed as protein to insure good fetal growth.[1]

Iron Requirements

Additional iron beyond that recommended for sedentary pregnant women does not seem to be required for the active pregnant woman. A 30 to 60 mg iron supplement, which is commonly found in prenatal vitamin preparations, will insure that maternal iron stores will not be depleted by pregnancy.

Water and Electrolyte Requirements

Physically active pregnant women will not likely be at risk of sodium depletion if their exercise is vigorous. Most people in the United States consume at least twice as much sodium as is generally recommended, since the reliance on processed goods in our diet is so high. Since sodium is not restricted during pregnancy and all pregnant women are encouraged to salt to taste, this should be sufficient for women who are exercising during pregnancy.

Additional fluids are advisable for pregnant women who exercise, especially if exercise is occurring where the ambient temperature and humidity are high. Consumption of 8 to 12 cups of water or other fluids daily is recommended to maintain normal body temperature and to support expansion of total body water which occurs during pregnancy. (This recommendation does not include soft drinks, coffee, and alcohol).

In summary, exercise brings about similar physiologic alterations in pregnant women as it does in nonpregnant women. Changes are most pronounced for the cardiovascular and respiratory systems and less marked for the musculoskeletal and endocrine systems. If pregnancy and exercise are combined, a doubled physiologic impact occurs. This fact suggests that if a prospective mother has not been involved in an exercise program prior to pregnancy, she should not be encouraged to begin one during her pregnancy, except for walking. Nutritional considerations are also very important.

With this general information as background, let us now consider the animal model and human clinical studies which have been reported and whose results may serve as a basis for selected recommendations for exercise during pregnancy.

ANIMAL STUDIES

Understandably, animal experiments have provided the most precise information available regarding effects from maternal exercise. Several studies using pregnant ewes with both fetal and maternal catheters inserted have produced similar results. Orr et al.[23] found that treadmill exercise in pregnant ewes did not change maternal mean arterial pressure while cardiac output and iliac blood flow increased. Emmannouilides et al.[24] found that fetal responses generally followed the maternal cardiovascular and pulmonary changes, including steady arterial pressure and increasing heart rate. The female ewes hyperventilated, producing a respiratory alkalosis with increased pH and decreased CO_2. These same biochemical findings were present in the fetus along with a reduction in PO_2. The authors suggest this hypoxemia was due to a reduction in the uterine blood flow during maternal exercise.

In another study utilizing pregnant ewes, Clapp[25] found significant detrimental changes in maternal and fetal parameters as maternal exhaustion approached. As maternal exhaustion was reached, the fetal PO_2 decreased significantly, maternal rectal temperature rose 1.4 degrees C, uterine blood flow decreased 28 percent, umbilical flow fell 10 percent, and maternal systemic lactic acid developed. Clapp speculated that fetal hypoxia was the result of exercise redistribution of cardiac output away from the splanchnic bed, systemic catecholamine release, respiratory alkalosis, and hyperthermia. These are factors which have been documented to reduce uterine blood flow by 25 percent.

Hyperthermia is another area of consideration of maternal exercise effects on the fetus. Edwards[26] conducted research concerning the effects of hyperthermia in animals. Induction of hyperthermia (body temperature of 40 to 41 degrees C) in mice resulted in maternal mortality, resorbed or aborted fetuses in 50 percent of the cases, and vertebral anomalies in over 30 percent of the surviving offspring. In a parallel clinical situation, Parker[27] observed a trend towards increased meninogomyelocele in newborn deliveries of women who exercised vigorously during the first trimester of pregnancy and who suffered heat stress.

Studies utilizing the pregnant ewe model have provided some of the best information concerning physiologic response to exercise. Lotgering, Gilbert and Longo[28,29] have published data on oxygen consumption, uterine blood flow, and blood volume as well as information about blood gases, temperatures, and the fetal cardiovascular system in these animals. A clinical extension of these and other data appears in a recent review by Longo and Hardesty.[30] Emphasis here is on the maternal blood volume, hypothesis of control, and clinical considerations. Again, the recent publication by Artal and Wiswell[1] provides over 180 references as well as a section describing experimental methodology which may be of interest both to the reader and the laboratory researcher.

HUMAN STUDIES

The effects of exercise on the human fetus are not as easy to evaluate as they are in animals. The assumption is made that the condition of the mother is not complicated by hypertension, diabetes mellitus, anemia, or other metabolic diseases, which in themselves affect management of the pregnancy. The few reported studies of exercise during pregnancy are limited to small numbers of subjects and all deal with healthy volunteers. In an early study, Hon and Wohlegemuth,[31] using a five-step climbing program, monitored fetal heart rates before and after exercise in 10 normal and 16 high risk pregnancies. After exercising, 20 of 26 subjects had no remarkable changes in their monitor patterns. Three of the remaining had minor changes and 3 fell into bradycardia, or an irregular pattern.

Using the bicycle ergometer, Pomerance, Gluck, and Lynch[32] monitored fetal heart rates before and after exercise in 54 normal pregnancies. A post exercise change in fetal heart rate of more than 16 beats per minute defined a suspicious test. Four of 5 subjects with suspicious tests had signs of distress during labor.

Hauth et al.[33] evaluated moderate exercise in 7 pregnant women who routinely ran 4.5 miles per week prior to and during their pregnancies. In the third trimester, nonstress tests were performed immediately after a 1.5 mile run. All nonstress tests remained reactive, although fetal tachycardia was present. All women delivered healthy infants at term.

Dressendorfer[34] studied the acute responses of the fetal heart rate using 5 trained swimmers who performed graded cycling exercise in a semi-Fowler's position at 32 to 39 weeks gestation. The fetal heart rate averaged 142 beats per minute before exercise and gradually increased during exercise to a peak of 149 beats per minute during the same time period. Dressendorfer suggested their findings portrayed a normal fetal heart response to dynamic work of submaximal effort. The aerobic exercise that raised maternal heart rate was approximately 80 percent of the maximum and did not produce fetal bradycardia or tachycardia.

Sibley et al.[18] studied the influence of aerobic swimming on levels of maternal physical fitness and the influence of each swimming period on maternal and fetal circulatory parameters. Thirteen low risk pregnant women were divided randomly between experimental and control groups. Experimental subjects participated in a 10-week swimming conditioning program while controls did not participate in any form of aerobic conditioning. Fitness levels for both groups were measured via respiratory gas analysis during graded exercise testing on a treadmill prior to and following the swimming program.

Experimental subjects were able to maintain their initial fitness levels, while the control group could not. Additionally, maternal blood pressure, pulse, and fetal heart tones remained for all subjects within clinically acceptable limits during the swimming conditioning program and treadmill testing.

In a retrospective questionnaire study involving 67 healthy, experienced runners who continued jogging during pregnancy, Jarrett and Spellacy collected data on prepregnancy health status, pregnancy and delivery information, and running experience during pregnancy. No correlation was found between running mileage and infant weight or gestational age. The incidence of fetal and maternal complications was low. A prematurity rate of 4.4 percent and one spontaneous abortion (1.5 percent) were reported. The information gathered suggested that jogging during pregnancy by conditioned runners is not harmful to the infant.[35]

Research conducted at Emory University has examined the clinical course of pregnancy and fetal and neonatal outcome in young women who continued to run or jog during their pregnancy. The majority of runners decreased their mileage as their pregnancy· progressed. Acute illnesses such as nausea, vomiting, fatigue, joint pain, ligament pain, uterine contractions, fear of harm to the fetus, and awkwardness were listed as reasons for a decrease in running distance. Also, training speeds decreased from 10.7 km/hr (5.6 min/km) to 8.0 km/hr (7.5 min/km). The mean increase of maternal body mass was 11.2 kg for runners and 12.9 kg for nonrunner controls. Length of labor in the runners ranged from 8 hours 20 minutes to greater than 20 hours, as contrasted to controls, whose labor ranged from 4 hours to 27 hours. Use of analgesics and anesthesia during labor and delivery was similar in both groups. All runners had episiotomies, except for those who had cesarean sections. Similar information was recorded for the controls. Infant birth weights averaged 3.39 kg for runners and 3.45 kg for controls.

Studies of simultaneous maternal and fetal heart rates during treadmill exercise demonstrated a transient fetal bradycardia in three technically acceptable tracings. This decline continued for 2 to 3 minutes at an intensity of effort likely in submaximal training. Recovery of the fetal heart rate to a normal range of 120 to 160 beats/min occurred after the 3 or 3 1/2 minute mark of exercise, before attainment of the target heart rate for the mother. These results suggest that moderate maternal exercise has no harmful effects on fetal heart activity.[36]

Other recent studies include those of Clapp and Dickstein,[37] whose data showed that women who continued to exercise at or near preconception levels during pregnancy gained less weight (4.6 kg), delivered earlier (8 days), and had lighter weight offspring (500 g) than those who stopped exercising prior to 28 weeks gestation. This latter group gained more weight (2.2 kg) but also delivered infants of smaller birth weight at the same gestational age than did the sedentary controls.

Investigation of thermoregulation during aerobic exercise in pregnancy by Jones at al.[38] demonstrated that mean resting skin temperatures increased whereas mean resting core and vaginal temperatures did not change. Core temperatures did not exceed 39 degrees C during weight bearing exercise stress of four aerobically conditioned pregnant women studied in a climate controlled environment during each trimester and postpartum. Heat storage (heat content/kg) was not increased as a result of exercise with advancing gestational age. The authors interpret their findings as being consistent with the hypothesis that thermal balance is maintained with advancing gestation when exercise prescriptions are appropriately modified for conditioned women.

The question of effect of exercise on uterine activity during the last eight weeks of pregnancy was addressed by Veille et al.[39] Two exercise forms, weight bearing (running) and nonweight bearing (stationary bicycle), were utilized. Results of study of 17 women show no increase in uterine activity as measured before and after exercise. Additionally, both maternal and fetal heart rates increased during exercise, with the fetal heart rate increasing significantly during the first 15 minutes postexercise but returning to baseline in the following 15 minutes recovery period. No change in maternal blood pressure was recorded.

In a larger study by Collings and Curet,[40] 25 pregnant women without recognizable complications underwent fetal heart rate evaluations during an exercise program targeted between 61 to 73 percent maximal capacity. The results confirmed previous findings by these authors of an acceleration of fetal heart rate in response to exercise. The exercise sessions consisted of 10 minutes of warm-up flexibility followed by 30 minutes of continuous aerobic activity. Walking, jogging, and stationary cycling were the chosen modes of activity. The exercise form was directed by acceptable prescriptions for the appropriate state of conditioning.

A summary of the results of several investigations is shown in Table 7-1. The question of alteration of fetal heart rate pattern in women with healthy uncomplicated pregnancies employing different exercise forms is unresolved at this time.[42]

A final consideration should be given to the work status of a pregnant woman. Chamberlain addresses this question in a recent editorial and raises several meaningful points. His general conclusions are that health care personnel pay much attention to diet and prenatal (home) environment but do not consider work outside the home. In the workplace, hazards of transportation, radiation, chemicals, boredom, fatigue, etc., also require evaluation and assessment of their role in the pregnancy outcome. Currently, advice by the practicing physician is overly cautious as physicians are uncertain of the basic and clinical data standards available to them.[43]

Table 7-1. Fetal Heart Rate

Author	Date	Pre-Exercise	During	Post-Exercise	Change
Dressendorfer[34]	1980	135–152	149±5	NR	Increased
Hauth[33]	1982	140–155	NR	155–204	Increased
Dale[36]	1982	133	108	131	Decreased–Normal
Collings[41]	1983	144	147	147	Unchanged
Artal[44]	1984	140	90	140–190	Decreased–Increased
Collings[42]	1985	140	NR	149	Increased

(NR=Not recorded)

CONCERNS ABOUT THE EFFECTS OF EXERCISE
UPON PREGNANCY

As shown above, the volume of research concerning exercise during pregnancy has grown the past few years. Many questions remain, as the studies have been performed on small numbers of subjects or have had technical or ethical problems associated with the research process. Furthermore, there are questions about application of results of animal studies to humans with regard to fetal effects.[45] Before addressing the recommendations for exercise during pregnancy let us first summarize the major concerns of most obstetric health care providers.

A summary of concerns about the effects of exercise during pregnancy include the following:

1. Fetal hypoxia, and specifically maternal hyperventilation reflects increased maternal oxygen demand during exercise, and the possibility that blood flow will be shunted from the uterus in favor of actively exercising skeletal muscle must be considered.

2. Generation of metabolic acids and alterations in energy and fat metabolism may also affect the fetus.

3. During exercise a pregnant woman may experience hyperthermia, which increases oxygen requirements and in early pregnancy is associated with neural tube defects, mental retardation, and seizures.

4. Fetal well-being and obstetric outcome may be influenced by repetitive mechanical stress of the gravid uterus on maternal skeletal and soft tissues.

5. As pregnancy progresses, orthopedic injuries may increase due to changes in maternal balance and softening of ligaments and joints.

More research concerning fitness of the pregnant female concurrent with fetal heart rate testing is needed to satisfy these concerns. Longitudinal studies of infant growth and development would also be informative.

With these concerns as background and with knowledge of the animal model and human studies, let us now examine the current recommendations for exercise during pregnancy.

Before giving these recommendations, it is important to note that agreement is not necessarily unanimous and that recommendations therefore carry no guarantee of favorable outcome or maintenance of fitness during the pregnancy. Legal discussions are beyond the realm of this contribution but should be kept in mind when describing prescriptions.

PRACTICAL RECOMMENDATIONS AND GUIDELINES

During the three trimesters of pregnancy and the postpartum period, hot baths, whirlpools, and saunas are to be avoided (particularly during the first trimester). While the mother should not begin a strenuous exercise program after she is knowingly pregnant, it is not necessary for her to make any radical changes in her ongoing program; rather, she should continue it. The standard classic Kegel exercises may be initiated at this time.[46] Finally, she should not take any medications during pregnancy unless necessary for treatment of medical illness and only as prescribed by a physician.

In the second trimester, unless directed by a physician, she should not resort to any type of special diet; exceptions are made in the cases of maternal hypertension and/or diabetes mellitus. She should avoid foods high in calories and low in nutritive value. A well-balanced diet is usually prescribed and when followed will be of advantage for both mother and developing fetus. A mother-to-be should also remember that exercise in pregnancy is not done for weight control but rather to preserve muscle tone, hopefully to make the period of labor and delivery easier on both mother and baby and hasten return to desired or optimal physical fitness following delivery.

In the third trimester she should avoid exercises which may compromise blood flow, particularly venous return (i.e., exercise while lying supine). She should avoid long periods of standing and/or lifting heavy objects. It is desirable to avoid those activities which might initiate uterine contractions and to avoid those activities which may lead to a potential imbalance by the mother, causing a fall. Activities which require a rapid change of direction, e.g., tennis or soccer, or activities in which the opportunity for a fall exists, e.g., horseback or motorcycle riding, are to be avoided. Ideal exercises which may be conducted throughout pregnancy include certain yoga asanas, swimming (at least until near term but certainly not after rupture of the membranes), and, most ideally, walking with good posture.

Depending on type of delivery and normalcy of delivery events, an exercise program may, and in fact should, be resumed as shortly after delivery as is felt comfortable by both mother and attending physician or nurse/midwife. Even before she leaves the hospital the mother can begin to restore muscle tone to abdomen and pelvic floor (puboccygeal muscles). Restoration of muscle tone to the latter through Kegel exercise will prevent the possibility of urinary incontinence or prolapse of the uterus and additionally enhance return to satisfactory sexual activity. Exercise also will promote blood flow and prevent stasis causing varicose veins, leg cramps, edema, and thrombus formation. The improved circulation will promote healing of traumatized pelvic tissues and strengthening of uterine and pelvic ligaments and tendons. While not scientifically documented, exercise may be useful in reducing or diminishing the postpartum depression which accompanies some pregnancies. The benefits of exercise have always been known to improve self-image, and this would be very useful for the mother during the postpartum period.

The major exercises to be avoided in the postpartum period are those which employ a prone knee/chest position. This position has been implicated in several maternal deaths and may be associated with air embolism or neurologic changes.

In May 1985 the American College of Obstetricians and Gynecologists (ACOG), in response to a number of requests from physicians and patients, presented guidelines for exercise during pregnancy.[47] At the same time, ACOG published two video tapes entitled "Pregnancy Exercise Program" and "Post-natal Exercise Program." While there has been great demand for these tapes, there has not been complete agreement on whether the guidelines or the video tapes for the patients meet the needs of pregnant women. A discussion of the opposing views appears in a recent publication.[48]

Guidelines and recommendations based on studies and reviews by Mullinax and Dale are given below.[49] Again, it must be emphasized that these are theoretical guidelines and must be individualized for the pregnancy under consideration. Like the ACOG guidelines, these recommendations are not intended to be applicable to all normal pregnancies, to complicated pregnancies, to women who are well trained, or to those who are poorly trained. They aim merely to guide and should not be construed as basis for litigation in cases of poor outcome.

The following are guidelines for counseling pregnant women who wish to maintain or develop physical fitness:

1. Contraindications to exercise during pregnancy are those conditions that increase the risk for disrupting the pregnancy or decreasing uteroplacental reserve. Those conditions would include pregnancy induced hypertension, diabetes, history of premature labor/delivery, placenta previa, threatened abortion, postdatism, multiple gestation, and smoking during pregnancy.

2. Exercise in the heat should be avoided throughout pregnancy. Hot tub and sauna bathing should be limited to 5 to 15 minutes;[42] water temperatures for tub bathing should be lowered during pregnancy.

3. Any activity that utilizes large muscle groups (running, cycling, aerobic dancing, tennis) should be decreased in intensity, speed, and frequency as pregnancy advances. Advising the pregnant woman to switch from running to walking or from aerobic dancing to swimming (weight bearing to non-weight bearing activity) would be an example.

4. Water skiing is to be avoided throughout pregnancy. Forceful entry of water into the uterus has been reported to cause miscarriage.[50]

5. Women are advised to stop scuba diving as soon as they realize they are pregnant.[51] Many factors related to this activity pose potential hazards for the pregnant woman and her fetus. These include increased risk of decompression sickness during pregnancy, teratogenic effects of hypercapnea and hyperoxia, and exposure to marine animal venoms that may produce adverse effects in the fetus.

6. Competition at an anaerobic pace is to be avoided throughout pregnancy.

7. Participation in contact sports is not advisable throughout pregnancy because of the dangers of falls and blows to the abdomen. This includes downhill snow skiing.

8. Racquet sports and those sports that require good balance and coordination (mountain climbing, gymnastics) need to be modified or avoided during pregnancy. As weight increases during pregnancy, the center of gravity changes. The resulting lordosis of the spinal column as well as softening of

ligaments and joints in response to progesterone may alter coordination and predispose one to a fall.

9.   Brisk walking affords the same cardiovascular benefits as running and is less stressful to the joints. Aerobic capacity can be improved safely during pregnancy by a regular program of physical exercise performed at least 30 minutes 3 times per week or more.

10.   For the nonathlete who wishes to begin exercise during pregnancy, prenatal exercise programs designed for low intensity of effort with a warm-up and cool-down period are recommended. These programs should be taught by qualified personnel with backgrounds in physical fitness and training. Each activity should be done gently over time with endurance and strength built slowly.

11.   Exercising to the point of exhaustion or chronic fatigue is detrimental to both the woman and the fetus. Pregnancy is not the time to work on a personal record in a 10 k race or to be training for a marathon.

12.   Pregnant women who wish to continue their weight lifting routines need to be advised to alter those exercises that may strain the lower back (i.e., dead lifts, bent rows, squats). Straining and using the Valsalva manuever to push heavy weight is not advisable. Many exercises using Nautilus equipment for upper body and leg strength building can probably be continued with modification (i.e., lighter weight, fewer repetitions with no straining).

13.   Postpartum fitness is improved when pregnant women enter their labor and delivery experiences in good physical condition. Following uncomplicated labor and delivery, many women can begin exercising again prior to the 6-weeks check-up. Gradual return to exercise should be emphasized with special attention given to fatigue levels, pain, and bleeding patterns. For example, if a woman resumes attending an aerobic dance class and a bright red lochia returns, the period of involution has not ended and physical activity should be curtailed until the lochia disappears.

The final but perhaps also the most important recommendation is that the decision to exercise during the course of pregnancy is one that must be made by consultation between parent(s) and the obstetric health team and should be based on considerations of maternal health, exercise form, duration, and intensity and how each of these factors may relate to fetal outcome. A major concern voiced throughout the years is the effect of maternal exercise upon fetal well-being. To date, no evidence exists to prove that a healthy mother guarantees a healthy fetus. Nevertheless, a mother who has a strong health orientation in terms of exercise and diet, who is a nonsmoker, and who does not consume large quantities of alcohol will certainly deliver a baby that is healthier than a baby born of a mother who continues to smoke cigarettes and consume large amounts of alcohol and/or other drugs and medications during her pregnancy. There is no suggestion that exercise during pregnancy is detrimental to fetal growth and development, nor is there evidence of reduced fetal mass, increased perinatal or neonatal mortality, or physical or mental retardation as sequelae to strenuous exercise performed during pregnancy.

Because of the newness of this field, we must await future studies to determine the impact upon childhood development, although it appears safe to speculate that the parents' health orientation will most likely carry over to their children.

A number of popular books emphasize Kegel-type exercises and yoga as being helpful to the mother.[52] Of importance is that the attending physician and/or nurse/midwife be familiar with these exercises so that he or she can discuss them with the patient, stressing why certain exercises will be helpful and why others should not be done. Whether the mother exercises strenuously or merely engages in daily recreational activity, the program does not have to be altered drastically during pregnancy. The pregnancy itself often serves to make the necessary adjustments in the exercise program. Exercise can be carried out alone, in a group, or with friends. It can be undertaken with the confidence that a healthy mother is the woman most likely to deliver and nurture a healthy baby.

REFERENCES

1. Artal R, Wiswell RA (eds): Exercise in Pregnancy. Williams & Wilkins, Baltimore, 1986
2. Cooper KH: The New Aerobics. Bantam Books, New York, 1970
3. Cooper M, Cooper KH: Aerobics for Women. Bantam Books, New York, 1972
4. Medical World News (Psychiatry Edition), p. 25, July 26, 1984
5. MMWR Weekly Report Annual Summary 1982, 31:128, 1983
6. Wirth V, Emmons P, Larson D: Running through pregnancy - not only is it safe, it may save your life. Runner's World 13:55, 1978
7. Wirth V, Larson D: Running after pregnancy - positive steps to getting back on your feet fast. Runner's World 13:45, 1978
8. Leaf D, Paul M: Giving birth to a new theory - is running o.k. while pregnant: Runner's World 18:49, 1983
9. Korcok M: Pregnant jogger: what a record! JAMA 246:201, 1981
10. Erdelyi GJ: Gynecological survey of female athletes. J Sports Med Phys Fitness 2:174, 1962
11. Jokl E: Physical activity during menstruation and pregnancy. Phys Fitness Res Dig 8:1, 1978
12. Zaharieva E: Olympic participation by women - effects on pregnancy and childbirth. JAMA 221:992, 1972
13. Zaharieva E: Survey of sports women at the Tokyo Olympics. J Spts Med Phys Fitness 5:215, 1965
14. de Swiet M: The cardiovascular system. p. 3. Hytten F, Chamberlain G (eds): Clinical Physiology in Obstetrics. Blackwell Scientific Publications, Oxford, 1980
15. Morton M, Paul M, Metcalfe J: Exercise during pregnancy. Med Clin North Am 69:97, 1985
16. Edington DW, Edgerton VR: The Biology of Physical Activity. Houghton Mifflin, Boston, 1976
17. Wilder E, Campbell L, Law C et al: Exercise and pregnancy: Cardiovascular changes during the second and third trimesters. Unpublished thesis, Emory University, 1986

18. Sibley L, Ruhling RO, Cameron-Foster J et al: Swimming and physical fitness during pregnancy. J Nurse-Midwf 26:3, 1981
19. Guzman CA, Caplan B: Cardiorespiratory response to exercise during pregnancy. Am J Obstet Gynecol 108:600, 1970
20. Knuttgen HG, Emerson K: Physiological response to pregnancy at rest and during exercise. J Appl Physiol 36:549, 1974
21. Artal R, Platt LD, Sperling M et al: Maternal cardiovascular and metabolic responses in normal pregnancy. Am J Obstet Gynecol 140:123, 1981
22. Porter (ed): Maternal Physical Activity Effects on the Fetus and Pregnancy Outcome: ICEA Review. 10(1):1, 1986
23. Orr J, Ungerer T, Will J et al: Effect of exercise stress on carotid, uterine and iliac blood flow in pregnant and nonpregnant ewes. Am J Obstet Gynecol 114:213, 1972
24. Emmanouilides GC, Hobel CJ, Yashiro, K et al: Fetal response to maternal exercise in the sheep. Am J Obstet Gynecol 112:130, 1972
25. Clapp J: Acute exercise stress in the pregnant ewe. Am J Obstet Gynecol 136:489, 1980
26. Edwards M: The effects of hyperthermia on pregnancy and prenatal development. In Wodlam D, Morris (eds): Experimental Embryology and Teratology. Elek Science, London, 1974
27. Parker G: Central nervous system defects linked to maternal exercise, fevers. Med. Tribune 18:3, 1979
28. Lotgering FK, Gilbert RD, Longo LD: Exercise responses in pregnant sheep: Oxygen consumption, uterine blood flow and blood volume. J Appl Physiol 55:834, 1983
29. Lotgering FK, Gilbert RD, Longo LD: Exercise responses in pregnant sheep: Blood gases, temperatures and fetal cardiovascular system. J Appl Physiol 55:842, 1983
30. Longo LD, Hardesty JS: Maternal blood volume: Measurement, hypothesis of control, and clinical considerations. Rev Perinat Med 5:1, 1984
31. Hon EH, Wohlegemuth R: The electronic evaluation of the fetal heart rate, IV. The effect of maternal exercise. Am J Obstet Gynecol. 81:361, 1961
32. Pomerance J, Gluck L, Lynch V: Maternal exercise as a screening test for uteroplacental insufficiency. Obstet Gynecol 44:383, 1979
33. Hauth JC, Gilstrap LC, Widmer K: Fetal heart rate reactivity before and after maternal jogging during the third trimester. Am J Obstet Gynecol 142:545, 1982
34. Dressendorfer RH: Fetal heart rate response to maternal exercise testing. Physician Sports Med 8:90, 1980
35. Jarrett JC, Spellacy WN: Jogging during pregnancy: An improved outcome? Obstet Gynecol 61:705, 1983
36. Dale E, Mullinax K, Bryan D: Exercise during pregnancy: Effects on the fetus. Can J Appl Sport Sci 7:98, 1982
37. Clapp JF, Dickstein S: Endurance exercise and pregnancy outcome. Med Sci Sports Exerc 16:556, 1984
38. Jones RL, Botti JJ, Anderson WM et al: Thermoregulation during aerobic exercise in pregnancy. Obstet Gynecol 65:340, 1985
39. Veille JC, Hohimer AR, Burry K et al: The effects of exercise on uterine activity in the last eight weeks of pregnancy. Am J Obstet Gynecol 151:727, 1985
40. Collings C, Curet LB: Fetal heart rate response to maternal exercise. Am J Obstet Gynecol 151:498, 1985
41. Collings C, Curet LB, Mullin JP: Maternal and fetal responses to a maternal aerobic exercise program. Am J Obstet Gynecol 145:702, 1983

42. Paolone AM and Worthington S: Cautions and advice on exercise during pregnancy. Contemporary OB/GYN Special Issue: The Active Woman. May 1985, pp. 150–164.
43. Chamberlain C: Effect of work during pregnancy. Obstet Gynecol 65:747, 1985
44. Artal R, Paul RH, Romen Y et al: Fetal bradycardia induced by maternal exercise. Lancet 2:258, 1984
45. Jopke T: Pregnancy: A time to exercise judgement. Physician Sports Med 11:139, 1983
46. Kegel AH: Progressive resistance exercise in the functional restoration of the perineal muscles. Am J Obstet Gynecol 56:238, 1948
47. American College of Obstetricians and Gynecologists (ACOG) Technical Bulletins on Exercise During Pregnancy and the Postnatal Period, 1985
48. Gauthier MM: Guidelines for exercise during pregnancy: Too little or too much? Phys Sports Med 14:162, 1986
49. Mullinax KM, Dale E: Some considerations of exercise during pregnancy. Clin Sports Med 5:559, 1986
50. Kizer KW, Point B: Medical hazards of the water skiing douche. Ann Emerg Med 9:268, 1980
51. Kizer KW, Women and diving. Phys Sports Med 9:84, 1981
52. DeLyser F: Jane Fonda's Workout Book for Pregnancy, Birth and Recovery. Simon & Schuster, New York, 1982

8 | Exercise and Pregnancy: Choices, Concerns, and Recommendations

Valerie C. Lee
Judy Mahle Lutter

More and more women now make regular vigorous exercise a part of their daily lives and wish to continue to do so during pregnancy and while breastfeeding. Many questions have been raised about the effects of maternal exercise on the health of the mother and the developing fetus.

In the last few years there has been a growing interest in researching the topic of exercise and pregnancy. When Melpomene Institute for Women's Health Research first compiled a bibliography on this topic in 1983, 40 items were listed.[1] In 1985, just two years later, a second bibliography included over 50 new citations, including a book entitled *Exercise in Pregnancy*. This increased research interest has already provided some new information. If we ask, however, what we have learned from all the research, we could answer, "Quite a lot," but also, "Not enough." One researcher summed up this dilemma when he noted that the research was still primarily physiologic rather than clinical. By this he meant we still need a good answer for the woman who asks, "Will I hurt myself or my baby if I exercise while I'm pregnant?"

175

APPLICABLE RESEARCH FINDINGS

Because of the limitations on the kinds of research which can or should be done with human subjects, animal studies will always be useful. However, questions about the transferability of findings from sheep or goats make research with humans preferable. For example, concerns about exercise-induced hyperthermia causing teratogenic effects in humans cannot be investigated with animals who use panting as the regulatory mechanism for cooling. A thorough review of what is known from the animal literature can be found in a recent book on exercise and pregnancy.[2]

Several reviews of the research on human maternal and/or fetal physiologic responses to exercise during pregnancy have appeared.[3-7] From these reviews it is clear that differences in methodology often result in contradictory findings. For example, fetal heart rate is often used as the dependent variable in studies of exercise during pregnancy. In response to maternal physical challenges, fetal heart rate has been shown to increase, decrease, or remain unchanged.[6]

Many categories of research are included under the general title, "exercise and pregnancy," with a wide range of operational definitions for the dependent and independent variables. Two general types of research are (1) laboratory studies involving physiologic measures of pregnant women during and immediately after exercise; and (2) surveys and case studies of pregnant women who exercise regularly. Both types of research have limitations.

Laboratory Studies

Laboratory studies can be divided into three types: (1) studies that measure maternal physiologic response to exercise, including maternal heart rate, blood pressure and temperature; (2) studies that look at the effects of maternal exertion on fetal behavior in which physical challenges are presented to pregnant women and fetal response is measured (measures include fetal heart rate and fetal breathing); (3) training studies that address the question, Can maternal fitness be maintained or even improved during pregnancy?

It has been difficult to extrapolate clinical applications from the findings in these studies. Despite a range of types of maternal exertions (e.g., ergometer, treadmill, step test) and a number of different maternal and fetal measures (VO2, heart volume, FHR, FBM, FM) no clear guidelines or recommendations for women wishing to exercise have been developed directly from these studies.

Laboratory studies have frequently involved women who were normally physically inactive. Those few studies which do involve physically active women[7-10] all have very small sample sizes. Thus, for physically active women the generalizability of findings is unclear.

Case Studies and Surveys of Pregnant Athletes

Case studies of pregnant athletes[11] do not tell us about the possible range of normal experiences physically active women might experience during pregnancy. Large scale surveys also have had methodological problems. The earliest studies involved elite athletes.[12,13] Patterns and outcomes of this group cannot be assumed to be similar to those experienced by the average athlete. Other studies have been retrospective. One survey involving recreational runners reported normal pregnancies, labor, deliveries, and fetal outcomes.[14] However, this data was collected retrospectively. A prospective study involving pregnant runners and nonexercising women found no significant differences between the two groups. However, sample size was small.[7,8]

Information is needed which is applicable not just to one or two women, animals, or elite Olympians, but to a wide spectrum of women of all ages and levels of physical activity. Such information should speak directly to the clinical concerns of women as to the safety of exercise for themselves and their babies. Several recent studies suggest that researchers are beginning to be sensitive to these clinical concerns.

RECENT STUDIES WITH CLINICAL APPLICATIONS

A study by Veille et al.[15] investigated the question as to whether there might be a relationship between physical activity and preterm deliveries. Some researchers have suggested that exercise during pregnancy increases the level of norepinephrine and thus can lead to increased uterine activity and possible early labor.[16] Past studies of working conditions and pregnancy have also noted a relationship between premature deliveries and working in a standing position late in pregnancy. Finally, Clapp and Dickstein found that there is an association between weight bearing exercise in the third trimester and early labors.[17] Veille et al. found that in a group of fit women in the last trimester of pregnancy there was no increase in uterine activity either during or following physical activity.[15] This held true for both weight bearing and non-weight bearing exercise.

Hyperthermia is another clinical concern involving physiologic measures. Hyperthermia has been shown to be teratogenic in laboratory animals. Elevated maternal core temperatures early in the first trimester have been linked to birth defects in human populations. The question is, Can dangerous temperatures be reached during exercise which would lead to negative fetal outcome? In a study done in Pennsylvania,[18] researchers recorded thermal response to moderate weight bearing exercise in aerobically conditioned women. During exercise it was found that core (rectal) temperature rose a maximum of .6 to 1.0 degrees C above basal levels but never exceeded 39 degrees C. Thus, for conditioned women at least, maternal thermoregulatory mechanisms appear to handle the increased heat production caused by exercise without hyperthermia.

The small sample size in this study (N=4) suggests that further research on a large sample is necessary before hard conclusions can be drawn. While these two laboratory studies involving physiologic measures did not find exercise to be problematic, an epidemiological study by Clapp and Dickstein[17] found that women who continued to exercise into the third trimester had lower weight gain, earlier deliveries, and babies who showed a lower than average birth weight for gestational age.

The causal factors behind these findings are unknown. The Clapp and Dickstein study is an example of a descriptive survey with a clinial applicability. Large scale natural histories of the actual experiences of women who exercise during pregnancy are useful in that they can reveal patterns which merit further investigation. In the absence of complete knowledge about the mechanisms involved in exercise during pregnancy, such descriptive studies provide some guidance for women in making decisions about lifestyle during pregnancy.

The Clapp and Dickstein findings about maternal weight gain and infant birth weights suggest a need for research about nutrition for physically active pregnant and breastfeeding women. A study conducted by Melpomene Institute[19] of 32 pregnant runners and 32 runners who had delivered their babies within the previous 9 months indicated that during pregnancy many women appear to expend more calories than they consumed. This was especially true in the third trimester. Following delivery these runners showed a consistent negative calorie balance.

In terms of diet adequacy most women were deficient in iron and calcium. While prenatal supplements corrected the iron imbalance during pregnancy, not all the women continued to take supplements postpartum. Very few of the women studied were taking calcium supplements.

In an earlier survey by Melpomene Institute of 195 women who ran while pregnant, maternal weight gain was the only variable to correlate positively with infant birth weight. Physically active women need to have enough calorie intake to ensure adequate weight gain while pregnant. If they are breastfeeding, infant weight gain will indicate whether they are receiving the appropriate amount of calories. Supplements at these times would ensure proper iron and calcium intake.

ORTHOPEDIC ISSUES IN EXERCISE AND PREGNANCY

Another area which deserves attention by researchers has to do with orthopedic issues associated with exercise and pregnancy. There has been one article on exercise and pregnancy by a physical therapist (Danforth),[20] and one by an orthopedist (Friedman).[21] No research has been done to assess questions about connective tissue changes, compression syndromes, or postural problems related to physical activity during pregnancy.

Orthopedic issues were included at the most recent Melpomene Institute study on exercise and pregnancy as a result of a presentation at the 1983

National Conference of Physical Therapists Specializing in Obstetrics and Gynecology. Those attending the sessions had concerns that had not been addressed in previous studies.

QUESTIONS AND CONCERNS OF PHYSICAL THERAPISTS

At the 1985 meeting of physical therapists in Orlando, a survey completed by 28 physical therapists attending a session on exercise and pregnancy provided some interesting information on attitudes as well as concerns. Of the group surveyed, one half worked in a hospital setting. Most of those who responded were either involved in a pre/postnatal exercise program or were thinking about starting one. When asked their reaction to women exercising while pregnant, all but one approved, on the condition that the women be physically active prior to pregnancy. All but two respondents felt exercise should be encouraged for most pregnant women. All agreed that there are some exercise programs which are better than others. Fifty-three percent thought that their reaction was similar to physicians, nurse-midwives, or other health professionals in their community. The 35 percent who felt it differed indicated that their response was more liberal; they felt the health profession in general was very conservative and often negative regarding exercise and pregnancy.

While these physical therapists approved of exercise in general, approval for specific forms of exercise showed wide variation. All approved of swimming, 78 percent approved of cycling, but only 53 percent approved of aerobic dance and 39 percent of running. A higher percentage (21 percent) disapproved more of running than of any other exercise listed. Almost 33 percent of the respondents indicated that they were actively looking for facts to help them decide what to recommend to patients.

Physical therapists thought that benefits could be grouped into two categories: physical and psychological. Under physical benefits, they listed weight control, strength, cardiovascular fitness, and muscle tone. Thirty-two percent also indicated that they felt being physically fit would be beneficial during labor, delivery, and recovery. Respondents felt that the psychological benefits of relaxation and improved self-esteem were also valid reasons to encourage exercise.

Most of the concerns were in regard to physical problems relevant to the health and safety of the mother and fetus. Those mentioned specifically were muscle and skeletal injuries, injuries to joints and ligaments, and problems with temperature and circulation. Physical therapists also expressed real concern about the lack of guidelines and adequate information. Fifty-three percent felt that the long-term effect of exercise during pregnancy would be positive. They also said the role of exercise during pregnancy would depend on a variety of factors related to the individual woman. These physical therapists indicated they would personally prefer to have additional information about benefits and problems before actively promoting exercise among their patients. The 3 guidelines they would recommend at their current knowledge level would be: (1) to continue prior exercise patterns; (2) to exercise sensibly; and (3) to seek guidance.

The Melpomene Institute studies have been designed to answer questions which can then be used by physical therapists and other health care professionals to provide guidance and answer questions which are clearly important to many women currently in their childbearing years.

EXERCISE AND PREGNANCY: A PROSPECTIVE STUDY

Methods

In the fall of 1983, Melpomene began a prospective study of the pregnancies, labor, deliveries, and fetal outcomes of 3 groups of women. Runners and swimmers who intended to continue to exercise during pregnancy as well as women who did not exercise regularly were enrolled in the study during the first trimester of their pregnancies.

Each woman completed a series of questionnaires. Data was collected on medical and exercise history, on progress of the pregnancy during each trimester, including information on weight gain, and on nutritional habits and exercise patterns. A fifth questionnaire was completed following labor and delivery. To monitor the health and exercise habits of the mother and the health and development of the babies, two follow up surveys were taken, one at 2 months and one at 6 months postpartum.

Participants were enrolled between the fall of 1983 and the fall of 1984. Exercising women were recruited through local and national running and swimming groups and through publications. Each woman was asked to identify someone who was similar to herself but who did not exercise to serve as a comparison. Nonexercising women were also recruited by word of mouth and physician referral.

The last babies were born in the summer of 1985 and 6 month follow-ups were completed by January 1986. A total of 177 women took part in the study. There were 110 runners, 32 swimmers, and 35 women who did not exercise. Data from 3 women (2 runners and 1 sedentary) who had twins were not included in the data analysis.

Among the 177 participants, there were 24 negative outcomes. These included 19 miscarriages (15 runners, 1 swimmer, and 3 sedentary women). There were 3 still births (1 runner and 2 sedentary women). One infant death was reported by a runner who delivered at 30 weeks. The child died 6 days later of respiratory distress syndrome. A 35-year-old runner's fetus was diagnosed with Edward's syndrome (trisomy 18). As a result the pregnancy was terminated in the second trimester. Overall there were no significant differences in the fetal mortality or neonatal mortality rates reported by swimmers and runners in the study and those rates reported for the general population of the United States. Spontaneous abortion rates for all groups were less than half the estimated rate for the general population of the United States.

After eliminating the data from women experiencing negative outcomes and multiple births, a total of 150 sets of history, trimester, and labor and delivery questionnaires were subject to computer analysis. These included forms from 92 runners, 31 swimmers, and 29 nonexercising women. Two postpartum surveys (2 months and 6 months) were collected from 120 of these women, 74 runners, 25 swimmers, and 21 nonexercising women.

Results

Parity, Age, Height, Weight

Participants in the study differed in terms of parity. This was the first pregnancy for 67.7 percent of the swimmers as compared with 42.2 percent of the runners and 27.6 percent of the controls. In other ways participants were similar. Their age at time of conception ranged from 21 to 39 years. Average age for runners was 30.4 years, for swimmers 29.6 years, and for sedentary women 29.9 years. Height ranged from 5' to 5'11". Average height for each group was 5'4". At the time of conception sedentary women were slightly heavier than exercising women, weighing an average of 128.7 pounds. Runners' average weight was 122.6 pounds and swimmers' average weight was 122.7 pounds.

Education

All of the women were well-educated, although more of the exercising women were likely to have completed 4 or more years of post-high school education (80 percent of runners, 83 percent of swimmers, and 58 percent of nonexercising women). Occupations varied. The largest categories were homemaker (15.6 percent of runners, 6.2 percent of swimmers, and 31 percent of sedentary women), and nonphysician health professional (14.4 percent of runners, 9.7 percent of swimmers, and 24.1 percent of nonexercising women).

Exercise Patterns

Almost all of the runners and swimmers began exercising before becoming pregnant (86.7 percent of runners and 93 percent of swimmers). The average number of years running was 6.8. The average number of years swimming was 13.2. In the 3 months prior to conception runners averaged 27.9 miles per week. Swimmers averaged 4,900 yards per week. The average number of days running was 5.3 per week and the average number of days swimming was 3.4 per week. These distances indicate that the women in the study were regular in commitment, but the sample is representative of the average rather than the elite athlete.

Prenatal Care

Most of the women were seeing an obstetrician/gynecologist (ob/gyn) for prenatal care (76.7 percent of runners, 74 percent of swimmers, and 62 percent of sedentary women). When asked if they thought their health care provider was knowledgeable about exercise during pregnancy, most said yes (69.3 percent of runners and 80.6 percent of swimmers). Among the nonexercising women, 64.3 percent said their health care person had made positive comments about exercise and pregnancy. Although not all providers were seen as knowledgeable, almost all were found to be supportive of exercise during pregnancy (91.8 percent for runners and 96.8 percent for swimmers). Hopefully the health professionals who were not knowledgeable would be able to give some guidance to their patients in terms of where they might find information about exercise and pregnancy.

Fertility

One important question deserving further study has to do with fertility and exercise. The relationship, if any, between exercise, menstrual functioning, and reproductive capacity for women is not clear. Melpomene Institute's research on exercise and pregnancy and on amenorrhea indicates that neither exercise nor amenorrhea necessarily prevents conception. In the current study few of the exercising women changed their running or swimming patterns in order to become pregnant. Ninety-two percent of the runners and 100 percent of the swimmers reported no change.

Physical Therapy Considerations

Discussions with physical therapists at the National meeting in 1983 encouraged us to include items on back problems and ligament strain in our investigation. Fifty percent of the runners, 50 percent of the swimmers, and 52 percent of the nonexercising women indicated that they experienced some back pain associated with pregnancy. Back pain associated with running was reported less frequently than back pain associated with pregnancy.

No swimmers reported back pain associated with exercise in either the first or third trimester. Six women in this group (18 percent) reported back pain associated with pregnancy in these two trimesters. In the second trimester, 37.5 percent had back pain associated with pregnancy. The percentage dropped to 28 percent in the third trimester.

Table 8-1. Back Problems of Runners

Associated with Running	Associated with Pregnancy	Both
1st Trimester 16 (17%)	19 (20%)	12 (13%)
2nd Trimester 19 (20%)	26 (28%)	16 (17%)
3rd Trimester 21 (23%)	28 (30%)	18 (19%)

For all 3 groups, the first trimester presented the fewest problems; the greatest incidence of back pain was found in the second trimester. Overall, the percentage of reported back pain are similar to the figure of 48 percent reported for pregnant woman in general.

Ligament strain was not a problem for the majority of respondents. Swimmers were least likely to experience problems; none of this group had problems in either the first or third trimester; 18 percent indicated a problem during the second trimester. Nine percent of runners reported problems in the first trimester, 18 percent in the second, and 9 percent in the third. A small percentage (8 percent) of runners also reported that they felt less coordinated during the second and third trimesters. Nonexercising women were more likely to report ligament strain in the second and third trimesters. Nineteen percent reported ligament strain in the second trimester and 20 percent in the third trimester.

Comparison of Pregnancies Between Exercisers and Nonexercisers

Outcomes

The overall results do not indicate any major differences in the pregnancies, labor, deliveries, or fetal outcomes of women who exercise vs those who do not. However, there do seem to be some differences in the exercise experiences of women participating in different forms of exercise. For example, runners showed a decrease in both distance and pace as their pregnancies progressed. Their average mileage per week in the first trimester was 21.2 miles at a pace of 9 minutes per mile. In the third trimester their average mileage was 7.8 miles per week at the pace of 11:45 minutes per mile. On the other hand, swimmers did not show much change in the amount or speed of swimming. Their first trimester mileage was 3.4 miles per week at a pace of 3,645 minutes per mile. In the third trimester they averaged 3.1 miles per week at a pace of 4,840 minutes per mile. It would seem that for women in this study, a non-weight bearing form of exercise such as swimming was less affected by the physiologic changes of pregnancy.

For those runners and swimmers who stopped exercising during their pregnancies, it would be instructive to examine more closely when and why they stopped. We shall want to know whether their decisions were related to maternal weight gain and infant birth weight. The interaction among exercise, weight gain, birth weight, and diet and nutrition are also important to explore.

Benefits and Problems

For both swimmers and runners, the primary benefit of exercise throughout pregnancy was psychological. The most frequently cited problems of exercising while pregnant for runners and swimmers was urinary frequency. However, in general, swimmers note few problems. One third or less indicated

Table 8-2. Most Common Problems of Pregnancy

Trimester	Runners	Swimmers	Sedentary
1st	Fatigue	Fatigue	Nausea & fatigue
2nd	Insomnia	Back pain	Insomnia & back pain
3rd	Braxton–Hicks	Braxton–Hicks	Insomnia & Braxton–Hicks

any problems in swimming while pregnant while at least one half of the runners experienced at least one problem. This same division is true in regard to problems associated with being pregnant in general. Runners are more like sedentary women in this respect. Tables 8-2, 8-3, and 8-4 indicate the most common problems for each of these groups.

Labor and Delivery. Similarities rather than differences between groups characterize the data from the labor and delivery and 2 month follow-up surveys. For example, labor and delivery occurred at about 39 gestational weeks for runners and 40 weeks for swimmers and controls. Swimmers experienced the longest labors, with a mean of 13 hours, while controls reported 8 hours and runners 10 hours of labor. However, these differences may be related more to parity than to exercise, since nonexercising women were more likely to be multiparous and swimmers primiparous.

Caesarean section rates were similar for the three groups: 25 percent for runners; 23 percent for swimmers; and 28 percent for the comparison group. There were few major complications for mothers or babies. Average Apgar scores for all groups were 8 at 1 minute and 9 at 5 minutes. Infant birth weights were also similar: 7 pounds 9 ounces for babies of runners; 7 pounds 3 ounces for swimmers; and 7 pounds 14 ounces for women not exercising regularly.

Most women in all the groups, including the women who did not exercise regularly, recommended exercise during pregnancy. As might be expected, exercising women were more enthusiastic than nonexercising women. Ninety-one percent of runners, 100 percent of swimmers, and 75.9 percent of controls recommended exercise during pregnancy. An additional 7.8 percent of runners and 20 percent of sedentary women recommended exercise with some cautions.

Postpartum

Child's Health. At 2 months postpartum, almost all mothers described their child's health as excellent or good. Most contacts with physicians were for routine checkups or common problems such as ear infections. All but a few mothers planned to breastfeed. By 2 months, 80 percent of the runners, 64

Table 8-3. Pregnancy Weight Gain and Weight Loss[a] PostPartum

	Runners	Swimmers	Sedentary
Gain	28.2	29.3	30.9
Loss	22.5	22.9	26.4

[a] In pounds.

Table 8-4. Body Image

	Runners	Swimmers	Sedentary
Just right	34%	20%	14%
Slightly overweight	49%	68%	62%
Overweight	11%	12%	19%

percent of the swimmers, and 76 percent of the sedentary women were still breastfeeding.

Mothers were asked to rate their babies on 7 dimensions characterizing their temperament. These dimensions included general activity level, regularity, distractability, and mood. On the average, babies were perceived as easygoing.

Mother's Health and Recovery. One sedentary woman felt her general health was fair, but all other participants believed themselves to be in excellent or good health. However, when asked if they felt fully recovered or back to "being yourself," only 53 percent of the runners, 60 percent of the swimmers, and 50 percent of the controls answered yes on the 2-month follow-up form. It should be recalled that exercising women believed that one of the benefits of exercising while pregnant was a quicker recovery. Fifty-one percent of the runners, 48 percent of the swimmers, and 52 percent of the nonexercising women also felt they had suffered some postpartum depression.

Case Studies

While statistics are instructive of overall problems which need to be further explored, several case studies may prove instructive for the physical therapist in clinical practice.

Case Study 1. C.F., a runner who also continued to compete in triathlons through the first trimester, reported back pain connected with exercise as well as back pain that she associated with pregnancy. In the second trimester she wrote that she felt her back pain stemmed mainly from her chair at work, but that it became particularly noticeable on a run. Her job also made it necessary for her to run at the end of the day, and she felt fatigue was a compounding factor. She indicated that she took it easy on days when her back was bad. Sometimes she found it necessary to walk and on particularly bad days chose to swim instead. She said she always just used "common sense."

This woman delivered vaginally with forcep assistance at 37.5 weeks after a 17-hour "extremely difficult" labor. The female baby was one of the smallest in the study, with a weight of 5 pounds 7 ounces. Apgar scores were 8 at 1 minute and 9 at 5 minutes and the baby was reported to be very healthy and active. Following the birth the mother reported that she felt strong and full of energy.

Three months later, C.F. reported a diagnosis of an irritated pubic symphysis which had occurred postpartum. Her physician's opinion was that the outer hip area had weakened and the inner part of her thighs had overdeveloped, a condition he felt was related to exercise during pregnancy.

He felt that weak muscles following delivery had led to a groin injury. The prescription was to do leg extensions with 5 pound weights 2 times a day. She was running 5 miles a day with discomfort. The orthopedic consultant to Melpomene suggested that the injury was probably related to running too soon after delivery, when the area was susceptible to injury. He suggested the patient add sit-ups to her exercise routine in her efforts to work through the injury and regain her prepregnancy level of performance.

This case exemplifies some of the changes which Melpomene Institute has observed during 6 years of research on pregnancy and exercise. Women seem to seek advice and cut back on regular patterns more readily in 1986 than they did in 1980. On the other hand, a too rapid return to activity based on the desire to look and feel "normal" may result in injury. Information on the possible problems of a precipitous resumption of regular activity may encourage women to give their bodies more time to recover following delivery.

In a telephone follow-up with this participant 2 1/2 years following delivery, she indicated that the injury had slowly improved with weight training. She felt she was back to "normal" after 8 months, although she said the groin area can still get tight. Before becoming pregnant with her second child she purchased a weight bench because she felt development of her whole body might prevent problems experienced in the first pregnancy. In the second pregnancy she ran until the fourth month but felt too uncomfortable after that time. She continued to swim 4 or 5 miles daily as well as to walk for 30 minutes a day. Her second child is now 3 months old and she reports feeling very fit. She has not experienced any problem with postpartum pubic symphysis pain, although she resumed exercise 2 weeks following delivery.

Case Study 2. M. V., a competitive marathoner running 80 to 90 miles per week before becoming pregnant, reported that she experienced severe sciatica and lower back pain following a 10-mile run at a 6:30 min/mi pace in her fourth month. Since she had experienced the same problem in college, she did not seek medical help but stopped for a few days and then resumed running a couple of miles a day at an easy pace for the next couple of weeks. She reported that the pain was relatively severe for 3 weeks. Because the pain varied from day to day as well as during her running, she did not feel it was necessary to totally discontinue. Walking, running slowly down hills, and stopping when necessary alleviated the pain.

When she returned to running she experimented with body position and found that leaning forward while running helped ease the pressure. This respondent reported relatively minor sciatica while running during the third trimester, although she had occasional pain with daily activities.

This woman was also followed in her second pregnancy. She did not achieve her prepregnancy level of performance between pregnancies and was running about 50 to 70 miles per week at conception. She reported that she was more cautious the second time, as she did not want the sciatica to reappear. She ran on grass more frequently and never ran fast downhill. The pregnancy remained uncomplicated by back or sciatic pain. Two months following the birth of her second child, she reported that she had some back fatigue but thought it was mostly due to lifting and carrying two children. She also thought it important to note that at 5′9″ she got back strain from working in spaces built for smaller women. She also said that she had never felt the back pain required medical treatment, including medication. She did convince her husband to give her back rubs.

A third participant, a recreational runner who typically ran 20 miles per week prior to pregnancy, reported sacroiliac pain if she ran every day. Running every other day seemed to alleviate the problem. She reported that she did not have the "fatigue-related" back pain which she had experienced with a nonexercising pregnancy.

In carefully reviewing the questionnaire data and conducting follow-up interviews with women who reported back pain, we did not find severe or lasting problems related to exercise and pregnancy. In 2 of the 3 cases presented, problems may had been related to higher levels of physical activity than that reported by the total sample. In each case the woman modified her exercise patterns and prevented a repeat occurrence during her second pregnancy.

One of the study participants, April Green, decided to pursue the question of back pain and pregnancy and is currently conducting a study as part of her masters degree in exercise physiology. She is in the final stages of completing data analysis of 17 women who exercised during pregnancy. She has been measuring parameters, including center of gravity, lumbar lordosis, and joint laxity at 3-month intervals during the pregnancies. She found that most changes occur during the last month or two and women are more likely to modify exercise patterns as a result. This substantiates Melpomene research on the entire sample with 63 percent of runners and 45 percent of swimmers discontinuing exercise in the final trimester. The average runner discontinued running at 31 weeks and the average swimmer at 32 weeks.

April Green's research also suggests that back pain during pregnancy is not always resolved following delivery. She feels some of this is related to relative lack of upper body strength, even in physically active women. She would encourage abdominal work in the postpartum period as well as overall strength training prior to pregnancy.

Studies like Green's, which objectively measure change, as well as continued follow-up of Melpomene participants over a 5 to 10 year time span should help answer concerns and questions of pregnant women and health professionals regarding the prevalence and persistence of back problems.

Practical Considerations

The Melpomene Institute studies, as well as those cited in the first section of this chapter, indicate that current research is beginning to provide information applicable to the clinician.

Further analysis of the Melpomene data will answer some of the important questions relating to exercise, nutrition, weight gain, and birth weight. Other issues to be addressed include changing exercise patterns during pregnancy, common problems of exercising during pregnancy and their solutions, major benefits of exercising during pregnancy, how and when to resume exercise postpartum, and nutrition for the physically active pregnant and breastfeeding woman.

Women who become pregnant will, however, want the most up-to-date information. It is therefore important to provide guidelines based on current knowledge. The individual woman should also be informed that hard and fast guidelines are not appropriate. She and her health care professionals will need to continue to discuss and probably modify exercise patterns as the pregnancy progresses.

Physical therapists have expressed particular interest in the area of prenatal exercise programs. As the demand for these classes increases, many physical therapists are involved in planning and teaching. In creating new programs it is often instructive to survey and evaluate what is currently being offered.

Prenatal Exercise Programs

As part of a Melpomene Conference on Maternal Health and Fitness, Melpomene conducted a survey of pre/postnatal fitness programs in the Minneapolis/St. Paul area. Twenty-two programs completed surveys. Pre/postnatal exercise classes were offered in a variety of settings, including hospitals, YMCAs, YWCAs, exercise studios, and community education centers. Respondents were asked to give general descriptions of their classes, including cost, length of classes, and length of sessions. They were asked whether medical histories and permission were required of class participants. They were also asked to describe the qualifications and background of instructors.

Almost all classes included warm-up and cool-down periods, and exercises designed to improve flexibility, strength, and aerobic conditioning. It was not always clear how such class components differed from other exercise classes taken by nonpregnant participants. Some programs offered information about pregnancy and taught relaxation techniques which would be useful during labor and delivery. These tended to be hospital-based programs which employed nurses or physical therapists as instructors.

The training and backgrounds of instructors varied, ranging from registered nurses to dancers and general exercise instructors without any special knowledge about pregnancy. Some instructors had received training through national maternal fitness programs or through various national groups which are attempting to certify teachers of maternal fitness.

Melpomene Institute suggests the following sets of questions to be used primarily by those attempting to set up a maternal fitness program and secondarily by those seeking a program to join.

Program Planners

1.   Why are you starting this program? Is it primarily for economic reasons?

2.   What do you know about the physiologic and psychological aspects of pregnancy and maternal health?

3.   What claims do you intend to make about the effectiveness of your program? What evidence do you have for these claims?

4.   What goals and objectives do you intend to establish? Will they include improved maternal fitness, preparation for labor and delivery, improved pregnancy outcome, faster recovery, and psychological or social support?

5.   What are your long term goals for participants? Are you expecting to facilitate behavioral lifestyle changes?

6.   How will you plan to achieve the goals you set? What type of program will you design? Would one class per week suffice to meet the program's goals and objectives?

7.   What types of exercise will you incorporate in the program and why? Will you include aerobic conditioning, muscle strength training, and/or flexibility exercises?

8.   Will your program include activities in addition to exercise which relate to maternal fitness? Will you provide nutrition education or stress management and relaxation instruction?

9.   Will you be able to individualize the classes? How do you plan to accommodate the individual needs and capabilities of the participants?

10.   What relationship, if any, will you have with other prenatal and childbirth education programs?

11.   How will you evaluate your program? What measures will you employ to assess how well the program has achieved your stated objectives? Will you determine and define your progam's effectiveness by simply looking at client satisfaction and attendance, or will you be able to measure actual changes in maternal fitness levels, pregnancy outcome, and lifestyle change?

Women should be encouraged to evaluate exercise programs before they enroll. Having worked with other agencies and individuals providing women with information necessary to make appropriate choices about exercise and fitness activities, we suggest that women look for a program with the following basic components:

1.   Warm-up exercises, to protect joints and muscles from injury and slowly increase respiratory and heart rates in preparation for aerobic activity

2.   Muscle strengthening exercises, to build and maintain tone and strength

3.   Cardiovascular conditioning exercises, to build and maintain aerobic endurance and improve cardiovascular and pulmonary functioning

4.   Cool-down exercises, to safely ease respiratory and heart rates to a lower level of activity

5. Relaxation techniques, to identify and release tension while further assisting metabolism to return to normal

6. Health education and discussion period, to foster a supportive atmosphere for the discussion of pregnancy-related concerns

We also feel that a well qualified instructor is the key element in a good program. Women should look for an instructor with the following qualities and capabilities:

1. Extensive background and/or certification as an exercise instructor
2. Training that includes information specific to pregnancy and childbirth
3. Ability to assess and monitor participants' health and fitness level, modifying exercise programs to accommodate individual needs and capabilities
4. Ability to teach participants
    a. to identify signs and symptoms of potential problems
    b. ways to reduce the risk of injury
    c. how to monitor their heart rates
    d. the importance of fluid replacement after activity
5. Sensitivity to the health education needs of pregnant women

Melpomene Institute would encourage women to survey programs in their area before choosing one. The following questions have been developed to help a woman evaluate available exercise programs:

1. What are the goals of the exercise programs? What evidence does the program director have that these goals can be achieved?
2. What is a typical class session like from beginning to end? Are participants required to periodically monitor their heart rates and to drink fluids?
3. What are the qualifications of the instructor?
4. Is a medical permit and/or medical history required of the participants?
5. What is the maximum class size?
6. Is there an opportunity to evaluate the program and instructor?
7. What is the cost of the program? Are scholarships available?
8. What is the registration procedure?
9. Are potential participants permitted to observe classes?
10. Is a postnatal program offered?
11. Is child care available? If so, what is the cost?
12. What medical help is available in the event of an emergency?

Finally, we would recommend selecting one or two programs and requesting permission to observe a class in each. Meeting with the instructor and talking with class participants should enable a pregnant woman to choose a program that is most compatible with her needs.

Because of the variability in quality and/or content of the programs offered, it is important that both provider and consumer proceed with caution. One of the most overlooked aspects of such programs is an assessment/evaluation component. Frequently, program goals are not specific or not well-articulated. Thus, it is difficult if not impossible to gauge the effectiveness of a given program.

In 1986, Melpomene conducted a two-part survey of participants in a national pre/postnatal exercise program. This program provided standard training for instructors and provided them with a standard set of program elements. Participants at 5 sites across the country completed one questionnaire at their first prenatal fitness class and a second at their final class session. The results from this study provide some insight into the nature and scope of prenatal fitness programs. The administrators of this program showed a remarkable sense of responsibility in authorizing this study, since most programs are not submitted to such scrutiny.

Slightly more than half the participants in this program were primiparous. Most began this program in the second trimester of their pregnancies. Few had engaged previously in any form of regular exercise. Aside from the class they were attending, few participated in any sort of other exercise. Indeed, most participants only came to class once per week and seldom practiced the exercise routines outside the class. Besides exercising, many had made other lifestyle changes during their pregnancy, presumably for better health. For example, it was not unusual for participants to indicate they had decreased alcohol consumption, were practicing better eating habits and/or had stopped smoking.

The two major reasons given for taking the prenatal exercise class were weight control and preparation for labor and delivery. These goals were somewhat unrealistic since there was not a major emphasis in the class on techniques specifically to cope with labor and delivery. In terms of weight control, the exercise routines were not vigorous enough to promote weight control and, even if they were, practicing them once a week would not be adequate. Indeed, the program designers only claimed the classes offered social and emotional support for pregnant women. Although there seemed to be some discrepancy between program goals and participant goals, the women in the classes were highly enthusiastic and very satisfied with the program and the instructors.

Maternal fitness programs might be most beneficial if they emphasized fitness for life rather than just exercising during pregnancy. Motivation to lead a healthy lifestyle is particularly high during pregnancy and women might be particularly receptive to learning how to incorporate exercise and good nutritional habits into their lives. This would mean a shift in emphasis from a narrow goal like weight control. Prenatal exercise classes might be a good place to encourage women to make this shift not only because their motivation is high but also because it may be the only place they have acess to the necessary information to make the appropriate lifestyle changes.

Women who have individually participated in sports such as running and swimming, however, rarely choose an exercise class. They are more likely to wish to continue their exercise patterns for as long as possible while pregnant.

Recommendations for Exercising While Pregnant

Information collected by Melpomene Institute suggests that many health care professionals and pregnant women would like some guidelines based on current research. The following recommendations have been developed after 6 years of research and discussion. These guidelines are meant to be just that—guidelines—rather than rigid prescriptions or proscriptions.

Each woman is different, both psychologically and physically. Each pregnancy should be evaluated on an individual basis. Women will want to discuss their exercise options with health care professionals, friends, and family. Once a woman has gathered as much information as she can on exercising while pregnant and has determined what her own priorities are, she will be in the best position to make decisions about her lifestyle.

General Recommendations for Exercise During Pregnancy

1. Exercise programs should take into consideration the medical and exercise history of the individual. The woman should discuss her exercise needs with her health care provider, especially if there are indications of medical conditions which might present problems (e.g., a history of miscarriage).

2. The woman should listen to her body. "No pain, no gain" does not apply to exercising during pregnancy.

3. The woman should expect some discomfort while exercising. She should learn all she can about exercising during pregnancy in order to have examples of normal discomfort and be better able to recognize possible medical problems.

4. If the woman has any questions about her safety or any unusual experiences (e.g., vaginal bleeding, elevated blood pressure, dizziness, or joint pains), she should stop exercising and consult a health care professional.

5. The woman should be alert to medical conditions which may indicate the need to change or stop exercising, (e.g., early effacement or dilation and multiple pregnancies).

6. The woman's attitude should be flexible. She should not have pre-set goals for exercising during pregnancy. She should be prepared to stop or switch to another form of exercise if she experiences discomfort which negates the positive aspects of exercise.

7. The woman should avoid an anaerobic pace. Her ability to compete will vary, depending on prepregnancy patterns.

8. The woman should receive psychological support for her decision, whether she decides to exercise or not.

9. The woman should be sure to get adequate rest. Exercise to the point of exhaustion or chronic fatigue is detrimental to both mother and fetus.

10. The woman should be sure that her nutritional needs are met. A balanced diet which results in normal weight gain is a good indicator that the

diet is adequate. Supplements normally recommended to pregnant women, particularly iron and calcium, are also important.

Recommendations for Runners Who Wish to Exercise During Pregnancy

The following recommendations are suggested for pregnant women who wish to exercise by running:

1. Because heat and dehydration can be serious problems, the woman should run in the coolest part of the day and in appropriate clothing. She should be sure to drink plenty of fluids before a run, even if she may have problems with urinary frequency.
2. The woman should take time for adequate warm-up and cool-down before and after running.
3. The woman should wear comfortable clothing. Stable well-cushioned running shoes and a good bra are important.
4. Some women find a lightweight maternity girdle offers support for back and ligaments. Maternity support stockings also help some women feel more comfortable.
5. The woman should be willing to modify her runs in terms of intensity, frequency, and speed. Increasing weight and fatigue may dictate shorter, slower runs and the elimination of running up hills or doing speed work.
6. The woman should stop and walk if necessary. This may be required because of heat, ligament or joint pains, or Braxton–Hicks contractions.
7. The woman should run with others if possible. She should always let people know when and where she is running. She should bring money in case she needs to phone someone to take her home.
8. The woman should pay attention to her posture and balance. She may want to experiment with posture changes that make her more stable while running. In general, she should be kind to her back.
9. The woman should modify or stop her exercise program if medical conditions dictate (e.g., early dilation, bag of water leaking).

Recommendations for Swimmers Who Wish to Exercise During Pregnancy

1. The woman should be sure the water and air temperature are comfortable. She should leave the water if she feels uncomfortable chilled or overheated.
2. The woman should take time to warm up. She should try doing some stretching on land or in the water. She should start off swimming slowly until she loosens up.
3. The woman should wear a comfortable swimsuit. Some maternity

swimsuits may be too heavy when wet for easy swimming. She should experiment with different styles and sizes until she finds something which she feels gives her support where needed and in which she can swim well.

4. The woman should swim according to her abilities. She should use moderation and be sure to breathe properly.

5. Diving or jumping into the water feet first, as well as water skiing, are not recommended.

6. If the woman experiences contractions, leg cramps, or joint pains, she should stop swimming or change her swimming style (e.g., use different strokes, kicks, and/or turns).

7. The woman should not swim alone but she should also try to avoid crowds.

8. The woman should modify or stop her exercise program if medical conditions dictate (e.g., early dilation, bag of water leaking).

In conclusion, the woman should enjoy herself. We have found that the most consistent benefit of exercise during pregnancy is psychological. Women feel that regular exercise during pregnancy allows them to have control over their bodies at a time of profound bodily changes. It gives them a chance to relax and helps them maintain a positive self-image.

Postpartum Concerns and Suggestions

Melpomene Institute has received many questions about the postnatal period. Physical therapists have had some concerns about long-term consequences.

Two months following pregnancy, 16 percent of the runners, 8 percent of the swimmers, and 33 percent of the comparison group mentioned back pain. Fifty percent of the swimmers experienced back pain while pregnant and the other fifty percent only mentioned problems postpartum. In the comparison group, no one who mentioned backaches during pregnancy had persistent problems, but 33 percent cited them for the first time. The participants' comments about back pain, however, reveal that this was primarily minor discomfort which the women believed to be related to lifting.

Most women are eager to resume their prepregnancy activities, including exercise, after the birth of the baby. However, some common sense precautions need to be taken. Very little research has been done on postpartum resumption of exercise. As with any question connected with pregnancy, women should discuss their exercise plans with a health care professional before making any decisions. For those women who have had casearean sections, it is especially important to consider physicians' instructions and wait at least 6 to 8 weeks before returning to vigorous exercise.

Information provided by participants in Melpomene's exercise and pregnancy research, especially in surveys conducted postpartum, suggest that for women who underwent uncomplicated vaginal deliveries the following recommendations may be useful:

1. If the woman had an episiotomy, she should probably wait until all soreness is gone, indicating healing is complete, before exercising vigorously.

2. Since the woman cannot use tampons for about 4 weeks, she may find it more convenient to wait until bleeding has stopped.

3. If the woman exercises and begins to bleed heavily and/or with bright red blood, she should give herself more time to recover.

4. Since her hormone balance is not stable for 6 weeks or so postpartum, the woman should be aware of continuing joint laxity.

5. Fatigue is a common problem for new mothers. If the woman becomes tired, it might be better for her to take a nap than to exercise. This is especially true if she is nursing.

6. Nursing mothers should remember to drink lots of fluids.

7. For women who are breastfeeding, good breast support during exercise is important.

8. Often, women are surprised to find they are incontinent after delivery. This can last for several months. The best exercises to correct this condition are Kegels. Women engaged in sports other than swimming or diving might consider wearing a pad or panty liner.

9. Often, the cumulative effects of pregnancy, labor, and carrying babies lead to back pain. The woman should watch her posture. Doing some abdominal strengthening exercises may help.

10. Adequate warm-up and stretching before exercise are important, as is a cool-down and relaxation period after exercise.

11. The woman should be sure to follow good nutritional habits. It is often difficult with a small baby and a busy schedule to eat properly. The woman should not be overly eager to lose weight. This is especially true if she is nursing, a time when it is to be expected that weight loss will be slower.

12. Scheduling may require some juggling. Many women find it difficult to make child care arrangements and/or to find the time for exercise in the early months.

13. The woman should relax and enjoy yourself. A brisk walk with her baby in a stroller or a pack may be all the exercise she can do at first. As she develops a routine and can schedule regular exercise, she will find such exercise provides important time for herself.

CURRENT STATE OF KNOWLEDGE; FUTURE DIRECTIONS

Further research on exercise and pregnancy is needed so that clinical decisions and advice can be based on factual data. Women who are physically active prior to pregnancy, however, will want information that they can use immediately. Given the precautions in the above recommendations, it would appear that for most women some level of physical activity during pregnancy is not physically harmful to mother or fetus. Current research does not reveal problems or outcomes which differ significantly from the nonexercising pregnant population. There is growing evidence that the psychological benefits predominate over physical benefits. Nonetheless, women who have experienced nonexercising and exercising pregnancies unanimously endorse the benefits of physical activity.

Some important areas remain relatively unexplored and should be the focus of new research. Nutrition as related to birth weight and nutritional adequacy of the mother has received little attention. The question, What kinds of exercise are safe for which women? can be answered by examining physiologic mechanisms affected by and affecting exercise and pregnancy. There is also a need for large-scale epidemiological studies of women who exercise while pregnant.

Longitudinal studies which follow the health history of both mother and child are important to measure problems and benefits which are not evident at delivery. Continued research and dissemination of information will mean that more women experience healthy, physically active pregnancies.

ACKNOWLEDGMENTS

We would like to thank Kathy Lohr for her research assistance and Vicki Novak for her editing and typing skills.

REFERENCES

1. Castor L: Pregnancy and fitness: a bibliography. The Melpomene Report, 2:23, 1983
2. Lotgering F, Gilbert RD, Long LD: Exercise in pregnancy in the experimental animal. p. 21. In Artal R, Wiswell R (eds): Exercise in Pregnancy. Williams & Wilkins, Baltimore, 1986
3. Lotgering F, Gilbert RD, Long LD: The interactions of exercise and pregnancy: a review. Am J Obstet Gynecol, 149:560, 1984
4. Marsal K, Lofgren O, Gennser G: Fetal breathing movements and maternal exercise. Acta Obstet Gynecol Scand, 58:197, 1963
5. Wells C: Women, Sport and Performance: A Physiological Perspective. Human Kinetics Publishers, Inc., Champaign, Illinois, 1985
6. ICEA Review: Maternal physical activity effects on the fetus and pregnancy outcome. Int J Child Educ, 1:1R, 1986
7. Mullinax K, Bryan D: Exercise during pregnancy: effects on the fetus. Can J Ap Sp Sci, 7:98, 1982
8. Dale E: Exercise and Sports During Pregnancy. Teach 'em, Chicago
9. Dressendorfer R, Goodin R: Fetal heart rate response to maternal exercise testing. The Phys Sports Med, 8:91, 1980
10. Hauth J, Gilstrap L, Widmer K: Fetal heart rate reactivity before and after maternal jogging during the third trimester. Am J Obstet Gynecol, 142:545, 1982

11. Dressendorfer R: Physical training during pregnancy and lactation. The Phys Sports Med, 6:74, 1978
12. Erdelyi G: Gynecological survey of female athletes. J Sports Med Phys Fitness, 12:174, 1962
13. Zaharieva E: Olympic participation by women: effects on pregnancy and childbirth. JAMA, 221:992, 1972
14. Jarret J, Spellacy W: Jogging during pregnancy: An improved outcome? Obstet Gynecol, 61:705, 1983
15. Veille JC, Hohimer AR, Burry K, et al: The effect of exercise on uterine activity in the last eight weeks of pregnancy. Am J Obstet Gynecol, 151:727, 1983
16. Artal RL, Platt L, Sperling M, et al: Exercise in pregnancy: I. Maternal cardiovascular and metabolic responses in normal pregnancy. Am J. Obstet Gynecol, 140:123, 1981
17. Clapp J, Dickstein S: Endurance exercise and pregnancy outcome. Med Sci Sports Exerc, 16:556, 1984
18. Jones R, Botti J, Anderson W, et al: Thermoregulation during aerobic excrcise in pregnancy. Obstet Gynecol, 65:340, 1985
19. Slavin J, Lee V: The expectant exerciser. Sports Nutr News, 5:1, 1986
20. Danforth D: Pregnancy and labor from the vantage point of the physical therapist. Am J Phys Med, 46:653, 1967
21. Friedman, MJ: Orthopedic problems in pregnancy. In Artal R, Wiswell R (eds): Exercise in Pregnancy, Williams & Wilkins, Baltimore, 1986.

9 | Childbirth Education Classes

Pamela Shrock

Teaching childbirth education classes is an art. The childbirth educator (CBE) is an artist who creates an environment for successful learning by including the expectant parents in the picture, by being ever aware of their fears, needs and goals, and by encouraging their active participation in the learning process. The CBE creates a class curriculum of up-to-date information and skills that are of practical and immediate use to the expectant couples and educates in ways that are creative, interesting and motivating.

Although both men and women make successful childbirth educators, in this chapter the pronoun "she" will be used, without intending offence.

THE CHILDBIRTH EDUCATOR

The childbirth educator comes from many backgrounds and disciplines, most frequently one with a medical orientation, such as nursing or physical therapy. Her choice of childbirth education as a profession usually stems from an innate desire to work with the childbearing population to enhance their childbirth experience by enabling them to emerge with positive feelings about the birth process, themselves, and one another. The enthusiasm she brings to childbirth education may stem from her own childbirth experience (whether positive or negative), from professional experiences with childbearing couples, as in a hospital or in labor and delivery, from the wonder that childbirth holds for her or from strong interest in teaching adults.

The CBE is neither a mother substitute nor a drill sergeant. Rather, she endeavors to help each parturient or couple to experience birth in the most meaningful way for them; the CBE uses special skills and techniques to assist in changing negative responses to the birthing process and to help women increase their confidence in their own ability, in conjunction with their birth

199

attendants, to cope with the stressful situation of birth. The CBE replaces fears and concerns—real or imagined—with factual information about childbirth and provides women with options and specialized skills with which to cope with the ofttimes stressful aspects of birthing their children.

Irrespective of her reasons for becoming a childbirth educator and apart from her knowledge and experience, teaching itself makes special demands on the personality of the CBE. Important qualities include being understanding of the feelings, fears, and concerns of the expectant couple, and having the ability to put herself "in their shoes" while respecting, accepting, and withholding judgement from all class members irrespective of their creed or orientation. She must genuinely care for her students by sharing her knowledge and time, yet not forget to take care of her own needs so as to prevent eventual burn-out. The quality of the teacher/student relationship is difficult to measure, but it is this rapport rather than the subject taught or techniques employed that is the essence of the education process.[1] No matter how specialized the system, how comprehensive the syllabus, or how sophisticated the visual aids, nothing compensates for this rapport, this spark that ignites the class and motivates the students to participate, share experiences, practice, and truly learn.

Being an educator, the CBE must be committed to becoming knowledgeable and remaining current in that knowledge. Her information base must be solid and broad, founded not on her own childbirth experience but rather on extensive clinical observation of the variety of ways in which couples experience and manage their child's birth. She must be thorough in her understanding of the cognitive, social, physical, and emotional aspects of pregnancy, childbirth, and the postpartum periods, even though she will not need to impart all of that information to her couples. She must research the resources of her medical community and be conversant with the intricate obstetrical practices in the various hospital labor-delivery rooms or family-centered maternity care facilities, such as labor-delivery-postpartum rooms (LDR) or free-standing birth centers. Likewise, she must know of the involvement, support, or lack of support or hinderance of medical caregivers, whether obstetricians, family practice doctors, midwives, or nurses. She must be familiar with the variety of medical technologies used throughout the childbearing year, and options in the use of medication and anesthesia must be at her fingertips.

Irrespective of whether she chooses to become certified by a recognised certifying organisation or plans to train herself, the CBE must have a working knowledge of the various methodologies in childbirth education, including the Read method, ASPO–Lamaze, the Bradley method, eclectic Lamaze, and psychosexual childbirth management.[2] Further, she must incorporate principles of adult education (based on the newest research), group process, communication skills, and the many physical and psychological modalities for relief of stress and pain.[3,4]

Skills and techniques related to physical preparation for childbearing women include physical exercise and postural re-education, relaxation, and coordinated expulsion and breathing techniques. The childbirth educator must comprehend the rationale or the reasons for the inclusion of each of these activities[4,5] and be able to perform them herself prior to teaching them to her couples.

Of equal importance, the CBE must create a nonthreatening environment for learning, in which the couples can try out new behaviors, incorporate new ideas and attitudes, and receive noncritical feedback and suggestions for improvement. The CBE, by understanding that people learn most when they actively participate in the learning process, encourages student input, incorporates the ideas of the couples,[6,7] and provides review, practice time, and feedback. By helping the couples set realistic goals she makes them aware of their potential and their possibilities, their options and choices, and the many practical ways that they can apply new information or skills to the birth process and to their daily lives.

ROLE OF EXPECTANT PARENTS

Childbirth education classes are distinct from other adult education classes in that they are geared towards couples or sometimes single parents-to-be in a group learning situation at a specific time in the life cycle. These couples are anticipating a new, intensely emotional and physical experience which will bring about a life transition from dyad to triad, from couple to family.[4] It is a time of imbalance, of change in homeostasis. Couples are faced with realities surrounding new responsibilities. They must deal with fears and anxieties and the possibility of pain. Needing support, they must rely on strangers in strange situations; recognizing their ignorance, they must sort out information and advice and come to terms with physical changes and emotional vulnerability.

The couples who attend childbirth education classes are not just training for a specific birth event; the childbirth education process encourages an acquisition of knowledge while attempting to dispel culturally-evolved fears and anxieties. Couples learn greater awareness of their bodies and related physiologic functioning and develop skills for both the childbearing process and for use in their daily lives. Perhaps more than ever before, they are called upon to become more aware of their values and attitudes, to make responsible decisions,[8] to develop new forms of communication for working less autonomously and more as a team, both with one another and with their medical caregivers.

Within the class situation, couples learn to improve their own lines of communication as they share needs and feelings with one another and discuss ideas with the other members of the group, and with their hospital and medical personnel. Most of all, they develop the courage to seek out that which they want and need in this maturational journey.

Generally, adult learners share similar characteristics. Because of time and energy constraints, the new information they receive must be relevant to their needs and must have immediate application.[5-7] They need to be encouraged to make their needs known and to set realistic individual goals.[9] Adult learners often equate learning with failure; because the fear of failure produces much anxiety, positive feedback becomes doubly important to them.[10] Most of all, they must be encouraged to take responsibility for their own learning. The adult learning process is different from that of youth; it must consist of varied stimuli and learning methods.[11]

PRINCIPLES OF ADULT EDUCATION APPLICABLE TO CHILDBIRTH EDUCATION

Adult learners, though wanting structured education with firm time frames and guidelines, also want some control over the learning process. It behooves the CBE to plan her classes with standard principles of adult education in mind and to recognize specific conditions that enhance the learning process.[14] Those principles include the following:

1.   Adults like to determine their own learning experiences and to feel that their feelings, ideas, and perspectives have value and significance.[5-7] Their fears, needs, and personal goals for their childbirth experience must be of paramount importance to the CBE in structuring behavioral objectives for the course and class series. An important responsibility of the CBE is to gather and record information about each couple's age, socio-educational level, beliefs, fears, and past experience with obstetrics or the medical world. The aspirations of and level of involvement desired by the parturient and her support person or partner is most important and must be respected.

2.   Adult learners draw knowledge from their past experience[4], a process which may create blocks to learning, such as fear of failure. The astute CBE can draw on the experiences of her students to illustrate information or move couples from concrete ideas to abstract thought (e.g., relating body responses to fear in the dentist's chair to the possible body responses to the "unknown" character of uterine contractions).

3.   The CBE must guard against including in her class series all of the information that she personally and professionally has accumulated. Adult learners have limited time for learning and home practice sessions. The couples attending childbirth classes are not preparing to become medical birth attendants. They primarily need only information and skills that are realistic and relevant to the impending childbirth, although some newly learned abilities, such as stress management skills, carry over into daily life.

4.   Active problem solving with practical answers and possibilities of tangible results motivates these learners.[9] Likewise, learning increases when couples identify the specific need for learning.[12] The subjects learn not only when societal and professional pressures require a particular learning need,[13] but also when the CBE provides revelant reasons and rationale for the inclusion of a skill or for the need of practice.

5.   Adults learn from the experience of others, so teaching in a group situation is most beneficial. The CBE must become very adept at group process; she must recognize that pregnant couples need physical comfort,

including sufficient space on chairs or carpeted floors with extra pillows for supported seating, reclining, or sidelying. Attention must be paid to proper lighting, temperature control, and convenient toilet facilities, as well as refreshments and break-time. Class members need time to move about, to communicate informally with one another, and break-time is an invaluable part of the classes. Communication is enhanced with added possibilities for exchange of ideas and resources or development of support systems and friendships if couples can recognize one another by means of name tags and class lists.

6. Emotional comfort within the group is afforded by the relaxed and informal atmosphere the CBE engenders. Her attitude of acceptance of all class members, her ability to offer nonthreatening and varied learning experiences, her involvement with class activities, and her providing time for small group interactions and discussions enable the subjects to learn from their own input and from the experiences of others in the group rather than relying only on information or direction from the CBE. These factors allow for the gradual reduction of the CBE's control over the class and for the couple's eventual assumption of control over their own learning.[15]

Above all, the CBE must recognize that people not only come from a variety of backgrounds with a variety of learning experiences, but that they also learn in different ways. She has the responsibility of providing varied and different learning experiences so as to include all class members, of maintaining their level of interest and of insuring that the learning process is fun and enjoyable.[11]

CREATING A CLASS CURRICULUM

In planning and designing a class curriculum, the CBE must write a syllabus or summary outline of her planned class series. She must ascertain the goals of the course based upon her extensive knowledge of the physiologic and emotional changes of pregnancy, parturition and postpartum, as well as her knowledge of hospital procedures and policies, cultural conditioning, and historically proven means of psychological and physical strategies for fear reduction, pain relief, and a more positive birth experience. Her goals must be realistic and of revelance to the couples with whom she will work.

When writing learner-centered objectives,[16] the CBE would be remiss if she did not investigate and then incorporate the personal goals and needs of the couples in her class. As discussed below in the section on teaching methods, adult learners are more motivated to learn if the information or skills presented are both revelant to their needs and are of a practical nature. Equally important, the CBE must not impose her own personal needs and goals on the couples. For example, if she feels that couples should not use medication during labor, she must not bias her classes against medication, for some couples may want or need to use medication in labor and may be left feeling guilty.

Table 9-1. Verbs for Writing Behavioral
Objectives

Analyze	Arrange
Brainstorm	Check
Classify	Compare
Compile	Define
Demonstrate	Describe
Discuss	Draw
Evaluate	Explain
Express	Formulate
Give examples	Guide
Identify	Interpret
List	Name
Outline	Perform
Plan	Practice
Recall	Review
Role play	Show
Simulate	Summarize
Teach	Work in groups to

(Knowles M: Adult Learner: A Neglected
Species. Gulf Publishing Co., Houston, 1978.)

Therefore, course objectives (intended learning outcomes) are written in the syllabus in behavioral terms[16] (Table 9-1). They fall into three categories: cognitive objectives, which emphasize remembering or reproducing materials that has been learned; affective objectives, which are concerned with feeling tones, attitudes, and emotions; and psychomotor objectives, which define muscular or motor skills. The function of these objectives is to provide direction for the CBE and to convey intent of instruction to the learner. For example, the CBE might ask the couple to list two reasons for backache in pregnancy (cognitive domain) and to demonstrate two exercises to help alleviate backache (psychomotor domain). Once the parturient or partner can indeed list the reasons for the backache and demonstrate the exercises, the CBE is assured that learning has taken place. Objectives, therefore, provide criteria for evaluation of the students and the learning process.

More importantly, objectives guide the CBE in selection of class content, teaching methods, and use of instructional materials or teaching aids.[11] For example, in order to discuss backache in pregnancy, the CBE must teach the couples specific vocabulary and basic anatomy of the curves of the lumbar spine. She must discuss the role of the abdominal wall, the efforts of stretching of the ligamentous attachments, and other changes that occur in pregnancy which affect the back. Some mention should be made of body mechanics and of the precautions to take when lifting. The CBE should discuss how to lie down and rise again from the lying position, and she should talk about the effects of increased body weight during pregnancy. To help the couples comprehend this material, the CBE might show or draw a picture of the lumbar spine and the changes it undergoes during pregnancy. (The Schuchardt charts are good for this). She may have the students stand and observe one another's spinal curvatures and discuss how they have changed. The CBE could use a model pelvis or demonstrate on her own body the increased lumbar lordosis and pressure points. To increase class participation, she could ask class members what they might do for a backache and which exercises they may have used in the past which might be helpful in reducing backache. (This method which is especially instrumental in increasing the involvement of the partners brings in past learning and experiences of the couples and is an example of the application of concrete past information to abstract reasoning.) In addition, the CBE could either demonstrate exercises mentioned by the couples or ask them to demonstrate for the class, or she could perform the exercises, explain their usefulness, and have the class actively perform the exercises while she offers feedback and gives affirmations or constructive criticism where needed.

Planning Class Content

In developing the class curriculum, the CBE must keep reminding herself of time constraints and especially of the limitations of the pregnant woman's attention span. She must curtail class content to include only what is needed to adequately prepare her class members for childbirth; she should not try to prepare them to be their own midwives.

An effective way to plan content is to ensure that each class begins and ends with activities that tend to reduce anxiety, e.g., warm-up exercises at the beginning of class and relaxation at the end. (For examples of class outlines, see Tables 9-2 and 9-3.)

All topics should relate to a learning objective. Content must be logically arranged, with topics flowing from one to the next.[10] For example, the CBE might first discuss physical and emotional changes during early labor, followed by a discussion of the feasible responses of the parturient and her partner. She might then teach specific comfort measures or exercises with attention given to the reason for the choice of that skill and what can be realistically expected to help.

In planning the sequencing of content, important points include starting with basic information and moving to more complex topics, from known facts to new facts, from beginning of a process to its conclusion, and eventually from concrete content to abstract levels of understanding, reasoning, and problem solving. For example, after discussing characteristics of muscle contractions of the uterus, duration of contractions, and shortened intervals in active phase of labor, couples might be asked, "What work does the uterus accomplish?" (A question which tests the couple's understanding) or "What other symptoms may prevail?" If they can't answer, the CBE might ask, "What may result in everyday life to one's body when it works hard over a period of time?" If they then answer fatigue and perspiration (appreciation of information), the next logical questions are (a) What could the parturient do to help herself? (ability to actively solve problem and (b) What could her partner do? (application of past information to present learning). This might be followed with role play of relaxation practice with support of partner, evaluation and feedback, and praise or constructive critique from the CBE.

Table 9-2. Class Outline 1

Class 1. Class introductions Reasons for coming Course overview Class goals Concepts of childbirth methods Historical overview Effects on pain cycle Effects on childbirth experience Physical and emotional changes Comfort measures Physical exercises Relaxation exercises	Class 4. Review of class 3 Questions Review of first stage; review of rules Review of respiratory progression Presentation of second stage Physical and emotional aspects Couple roles Expulsion techniques Review of relaxation techniques

Class 2. Review
Questions regarding past infor-
mation
Review of physical exercises
Review of relaxation awareness
Practice drill
Overview of labor and delivery
Early labor
Physical and emotional changes
Role of parturient
Role of partner/support person
Introduction of respiratory tech-
niques
	Class 5. Review of all techniques for labor
	Role play situations
	Review of entire labor
	    Hospital admission
	    Delivery procedures
	    Couple roles
	Movie or slides
	Discussion of third stage
	Variations of second stage
	Anesthesia
	Appearance of newborn
	Discussion of immediate postpartum
	Physical & emotional changes

Class 3. Review and feedback Review of relaxation skills Review of respiratory basics Relaxation in different position Active labor and transition Respiratory progression for labor Variations of first stage Back labor Medication Induction, augmentation Fetal monitoring	Class 6. Review of all techniques and labor Discussion of postpartum in depth Physical recovery Emotional needs and feelings of new parents Newborn needs Postpartum exercise

An often overlooked aspect of learning in a childbirth class is the exchange of ideas between couples. To this end, the CBE must provide the means to increase group process throughout the classes and help couples become acquainted with one another by sharing ideas in small group discussions. Couples especially value informal time for socializing with one another during breaks. Couples give and receive much needed support from one another, and the ability to feel a commonality of purpose and experience provides emotional sustenance.[9]

An important consideration is to summarize briefly the content at the end of each topic, and to reserve time for class discussion or questions before proceeding to the next topic. An overall summary at the end of each class helps to bring closure to the various facets of that evening's learning. The CBE might also take time at the end of class to recommend additional outside reading and ideas for practice of relaxation or breathing techniques. A brief overview of

Table 9-3. Class Outline 2

Class 1	Class introductions; instructor and class members
	Class information; "housekeeping"
	Historical overview of obstetrics/childbirth education
	Aims of childbirth preparation
	Areas of preparation (physical, emotional, intellectual)
	How techniques work
	Benefits of childbirth preparation
	Misconceptions
	Couple role, medical team roles
	BREAK
	Anatomy of pregnancy, fetal development
	Physical and emotional changes in pregnancy
	Introduction to breastfeeding
	Comfort measures and body mechanics
	Prenatal exercises
	Relaxation awareness exercises
	Closure, practice
	Overview of following week
Class 2	Warm-ups and introductions
	Review of prenatal exercise
	Additional exercises
	Review of awareness exercises
	Progressive relaxation exercises
	Conscious control and feedback
	Touch relaxation
	BREAK
	Review of vocabulary and anatomy
	Function of uterus
	Overview of labor
	Details of early phase of labor
	Role of couple
	Breathing basics
	Slow-paced breathing
	Summary and closure
	Homework practice
	Overview of following week

some of the content of the next class adds a sense of continuity and creates an anticipation of further progress.

TEACHING METHODS

Having decided on class content, the CBE has the responsibility of helping students achieve valid learning objectives through a combination of teaching methods and activities. She should select different kinds of appropriate instructional materials and media and arrange them for their most effective use.[11]

People learn in a variety of ways; learning involves different perceptions through various sensory modes. Some cognitive learners acquire and retain information by hearing words, listening to a lecture, or in discussion with peers. Others need to see words written in texts, on the blackboard, in handouts, or summarized on a chart.

Reflective learners use sight for increased learning retention and enjoy illustrations, charts, photographs, models, demonstrations of exercises, or observing activities or skills. Auditory learners may listen to words but respond to rhythms, cadence, and music from records, tape cassettes, or combined audio-visual presentations of slides and narration. Tactile learners learn by touch, by experiencing body movements, or by feeling the circles of dilatation charts.

To master a skill, most learners need to not only hear the description of the technique, but to actually perform the exercise. For example, in mastering breathing techniques, a combination of sensory perceptions may be needed by learners; students may need to hear a description of how to do the exercise, watch a demonstration of the breathing, hear the rhythm, and feel the movement of the chest through repeated practice.

Research in learning has determined that greater retention of material results from a combination of visual and auditory stimuli and from students' actual participation in learning activities. A Chinese proverb explains it thus:

> *That which I hear, I forget*
> *That which I see, I remember*
> *That which I do, I understand*

The astute CBE, therefore, recognizes that she must include many varied teaching methods as well as sensory, visual, auditory, tactile, proprioceptive, and kinesthetic stimuli. By means of different types of instructional materials she enhances the learning capabilities of her students.

The most effective learning is direct learning through sensory contact and participation with reality. Sometimes direct learning is not feasible, and in the case of childbirth education, this is often the case. For example, one cannot observe the growth of the fetus in utero or witness the process of birth. The CBE will often use spoken words (abstract symbols of reality) as in a lecture or discussion or presentation of issues for clarification, or the written word, as in handouts or readings from books, magazine articles, or journals. Lecture is a recognized form of teaching but is not the most effective. The creative CBE must recognize the importance of involving her students in their learning process and must select teaching methods that encourage low teacher involvement and high learner involvement.[7] Such methods include small group discussion, brainstorming, role-playing, role reversal (a method most useful for involving the partner and increasing his appreciation of the woman's experience), labor rehearsal, debate and problem solving, practice of techniques, and role exchange, in which the students do the teaching. These forms of active participation must be interwoven into the classes along with information presented by the childbirth educator.

Another important factor that must be included is the CBE's evaluation of her students. Often this is immediate, as in the students' demonstration of a newly learned skill. At other times it needs to be organized in the form of review in the following class. The CBE should not make the mistake of using only question and answer to review or evaluate information, but should do so in the form of student teaching in which students teach previously learned information, brainstorming in small groups, or formulating a birth plan and presenting it to a physician. Such a plan might incorporate various facets of hospital procedures which the couple wish to discuss. Evaluation enables the CBE to receive feedback on the level of the student's comprehension of material or performance of skill, but more importantly can alert her of the need to describe again information learned or correct inconsistencies.

Instructional Materials

An excellent means of making information more concrete, teachable,[5] and understandable is through the use of representation of reality or by instructional materials and media. If the students cannot observe reality directly, they can learn through vicarious representations of reality provided by teaching aids and instructional materials. Instructional materials that make learning more dynamic and realistic not only foster the learning process but allow students to make more effective use of limited class time.

Instructional materials extend the limitations of human experience and the limits of the classroom. Not many couples have seen the inside of the labor suite nor have they been exposed to the dramatic events of the birth process. With slides, movies, birth atlases, models of reproductive organs, pictorial illustrations of hospital procedures, hospital tours, and dramatizations of expulsion, the CBE can enhance her students' perception and learning.

From abstract words written on blackboard or flip chart to detailed illustrations in birth atlases or a simple demonstration of effacement and dilatation by means of a polo-necked sweater and the CBE's fist, instructional materials provide meaningful illustrations that clarify and supplement primary sources of information. They decrease misconception, as when they are used to explain the mechanism of expulsion through the use of models of the fetus and pelvis or through charts depicting cardinal movements during labor.

Material can be simplified or amplified by sequential teaching. The CBE might start by presenting the basics using a pelvic model. She might then broaden her presentation through progressive illustrations of the changes of pregnancy as shown on Schuchardt charts. The CBE might demonstrate postural changes with her own body, or draw stick-figures on a blackboard to illustrate pelvic tilt exercises. Or she may have her students perform postural correction exercises to music.

The CBE can maintain interest and add drama by demonstrating effacement and dilatation using a knitted uterus with fetal model or large grapefruit, or cardboard pelvis and baby to illustrate cardinal movements through the pelvis.

The use of music and the CBE's voice can stimulate and motivate students to participate during exercise practice, especially if the CBE performs the exercises along with the class.

Instructional materials help in summarizing and reviewing material. This may be done by listing transition symptoms on chart or on blackboard from student input, or listing goody-bag uses from actual contents presented.

It is important to realize, however, that no single medium or method is best for learning any one subject, acquiring a skill, or developing desirable attitudes. A variety of media can be effective in any number of areas. The most important consideration is whether the materials are consistent with and work well with the objective and content for which they were chosen.

The following questions may help the CBE to select instructional materials: Will the instructional aids enhance, clarify, summarize, or simplify class material? Are they cost-effective or just a gimmick and wasteful of time? Are they up-to-date and will they stimulate learning?

The CBE would benefit by ascertaining the advantages and disadvantages of the variety of instructional materials and then by including them judiciously into her class curriculum.

THE CHILDBIRTH EDUCATOR AS PROFESSIONAL

Besides the CBE's many roles as service provider, ongoing learner, group leader, creative instructor, imparter of information, she is also a professional businesswoman. As such she must maintain records of her students, her activities, her expenses and her income.

Class Records

Any system of record keeping should be simple, functional, and require minimal effort. A master card (4" × 6" or 5" × 8") filed in a metal box or a chart with the registration form with all it's information about names, addresses, phone numbers, ages, occupations, birth attendants, (with addresses and phone numbers), number of pregnancy, number of children, information about past obstetric history, desire to breastfeed, name of pediatrician, and even reasons for attending classes should be kept. (The CBE should keep enough material to allow her to be acquainted with the class members and their history and to make her aware of problem areas and progress through the series.) These cards are a means to verify payment, and if a referral note is obtained from the physician, to be reminded of any medical condition.

On each card records can be kept of student attendance, student progress through the classes, including positive and negative feelings, attitudes and improvements, or problems that arise, such as specific pains (i.e., sciatic nerve involvement) or specific conditions (i.e., toxemia). The cards can also be used to record special requests. Final night comments may include prognosis or possible need to contact the student for review class. After birth records of labor, details about the baby, and any follow-up contact, such as attendance at class reunions, can be added or problems reported.

Permanent files enable the CBE to contact former students to inform them of baby massage classes, interesting meetings about child care, or for networking for support groups. Stored alphabetically, they can be available for future follow-up, when couples call for refresher courses for their next baby. Also, in these days of litigation, it may be advisable to maintain records to the length of the statute of limitations of the state in which the CBE practices.

CONCLUSION

The CBE is a professional with a deepseated caring for childbearing populations and whose background is generally of medical orientation (physical therapist, nurse). She has broadened her education of obstetrics and gynecology to include many facets of adult education, including group process, principles of learning, teaching techniques, and the use of audio-visual materials. She must carefully organize her class series to meet the needs and goals of the childbearing population with whom she will work so that the learning experience will be a practical and fun one.

REFERENCES

1. Kitzinger S: Education and Counseling for Childbirth. Schocken Books, New York, 1977
2. Bean C: Methods of Childbirth. Doubleday, New York, 1972
3. Humenick S (ed): Expanding Horizons in Childbirth Education. ASPO-Lamaze, Arlington, Virginia, 1983
4. Ewy, D (ed): Expanding Horizons in Childbirth Education. ASPO-Lamaze, Arlington, Virginia, 1984
5. Pine G, Horne P: Principles and Conditions for Learning in Adult Education. Adult Leadership, Oct 1969.
6. Knowles M: Adult Learner: A Neglected Species. Gulf Publishing, Houston, 1978
7. Knowles M: The Modern Practice of Adult Education from Pedagogy to Androgogy. Association Press, Houston, 1980
8. Hassid P: Textbook for Childbirth Educators. Harper & Row, London, 1984
9. Tarnow, K: Working with Adult Learners. Nurse educator. Sept/Oct 1979
10. Long H: Adult Learning: Research and Practice. The Adult Education Co, 1983
11. Shrock P, Bunin N, Shearer M: Directory of Instructional Materials in Childbirth and New Parent Education. 2nd Edition. Berkeley, California. 1982
12. Jarvis P: Adult and Continuing Education, Theory and Practice. Nichols Publishing, 1983
13. Taylor B, Verble M: Instructional Skills for Health Care Educators. University of Kentucky Press, 1984
14. Thompson JB: Selected principles of teaching and learning applied to nurse-widwifery clinical education. Journal of Nurse-Midwifery. 28:1, 1983
15. Verdiun J, Miller H, Greer C: Adults Teaching Adults. Learning Concepts, 1977
16. Mager R: Preparing Instructional Objectives. Fearson Publications, Palo Alto, California, 1962

SELECTED READINGS FOR TEACHING AIDS

Anderson RL: Selecting and Developing Media for Instruction. Van Nostrand Rheinhold, Cincinatti, 1976

Brown, Lewis, Harcleroad: A-V Instruction: Technology: Media and Methods. McGraw-Hill, New York, 1973

Brown R: Educational Media: Competency Based Approach. Charles Merrill, Columbus, Ohio, 1972

Bullough R: Creating Instructional Materials. Charles Merrill, Columbus, Ohio, 1974

Clark C: Using Instructional Objectives in Teaching. Scott Foresman & Co, Glenview, Illinois, 1972

Dale, E: Audio-visual Methods of Teaching. Holt, Rinehart & Winston, New York, 1969

Erickson C, Carl D: Fundamentals of Teaching with Audiovisual Technology. Macmillan, New York, 1972

Gagne R, Briggs L: Principles of Instructional Design. Prentice Hall, Englewood Cliffs, New Jersey, 1974

Haney J, Ullmer E: Educational Media and the Teacher, Brown & Co, Dubuque, 1970

Jamison DT, Klees SJ, Wells SJ: Cost of Educational Media-Guidelines for Planning and Evaluation. Sage Publications, Beverly Hills, 1978

Kemp, JE: Planning and Producing Audiovisual Materials. 4th Ed. Harper & Row, New York, 1980

Kinney L, Dresden K: Better Learning Through Current Materials. Stanford University Press, Stanford, California, 1952

Reiser RA, Gagne RM: Selecting Media for Instruction. Educational Technical Publisher, Englewood Cliffs, New Jersey, 1983

Shrock, P, Ellis J, Bunnin N: Directory of Instructional Materials in Childbirth and New Parent Education. 2nd. Ed. Berkeley, 1982

Smith H., Nagel T: Instructional Media and Learning Process. Charles Merrill, Columbus, 1972

Wittich W, Schuller C: Instructional Technology: Its Nature and Use. 4th Ed. Harper & Row, New York, 1979

Woodbury M: Selecting Materials for Instruction: Subject Areas and Implementation. Littleton, 1980

Zirber L: Spurs to Creative Teaching. Putnam, New York, 1959

APPENDIX
Childbirth Education Resource List

Audio Visual Catalogs

Directory of Instructional Materials in Childbirth & New Parent Education

Blackwell Scient. Publishers
52 Beacon Street
Boston, MA 02108

Whole Birth Catalogue

Janet Isaacs Ashford
14230 Elva Ave.
Saratoga, CA 95070

March of Dimes

1275 Mamaroneck Ave.
White Plains, NY 10605

Magazines

Childbirth Educator

575 Lexington Ave.
New York, NY 10022

American Baby Magazine
Childbirth Educator

575 Lexington Ave.
New York, NY 10022

Lamaze Parents' Magazine

ASPO-Lamaze
1840 Wilson Blvd
Arlington, VA 22201

Birth Journal

Blackwell Public
52 Beacon St.
Boston, MA 02108

Movies (Catalog Available)

Polymorph Films

118 South Street
Boston, MA 02111

Center Films

1103 N. El Camino Ave.
Hollywood, CA 90038

Parenting Pictures

121 N.W. Crystal Street
Crystal River, FL 32629

Slides

Babes

59 Berens Drive
Kentfield, CA 94904

Artemis

Box 3147
Stamford, CN 06905

Educational Graphics

1315 Norwood
Boulder, CO 80302

Charts/Models/Slides

Childbirth Graphics

Box 17025
Irondequoit Post Office
Rochester NY 14617

Pharmaceutical Firms

Ross Laboratories
(Booklets & Visual Aids)

Columbus, OH 43216

Hollister Co.
(Samples)

212 E. Chicago Ave.
Chicago, IL 60611

Foreign Language

Womens' International News Service
(Illustrations in English, Spanish, French, Arabic)

187 Grant Street
Lexington, MA 02173

This is only a partial list of resources. For a more extensive list see *Directory of Instructional Materials*.

Appendices*

Elizabeth Noble

The following are materials for instructing women in postpartum and prenatal exercise.

SUMMARY OF ESSENTIAL EXERCISES FOLLOWING CAESAREAN BIRTH

Commence as soon as you recover from the anesthetic. Do each exercise twice to start, progressing at your own pace through the phases. Relax and breathe deeply between each exercise. The sequence can be repeated in reverse order.

Phase I

    1. Breathing exercises. Upper chest, mid-chest, diaphragmatic with abdominal wall tightening.

    2. Huffing. These two are very important if general anesthesia was used.

    3. Foot exercises. Bend, stretch, rotate.

    4. Leg-bracing. Tense and relax legs. Continue these for as long as you are confined to bed.

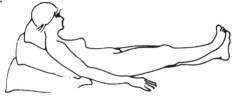

---

* The appendices are modified from Noble E: Essential Exercises for the Childbearing Years. Houghton Mifflin, Boston, 1982.

215

Phase II

5. Bending and straightening alternate knee.

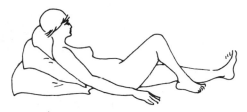

6. Pelvic-Rocking. Combine with pelvic floor contractions.

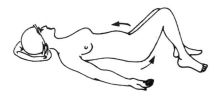

Before standing: Bend knees; use arms to turn toward edge of bed. Sit first and swing feet a few times. Brace abdominal muscles as you stand upright.

Posture check.

Phase III

7. Bridge and twist.   8. Reach to the knees.

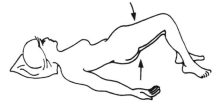 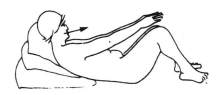

Phase IV

Check for separation of the recti muscles. Check stopping and starting of urine flow.

9. Straight curl-up.   10. Leg-sliding.

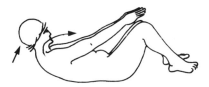 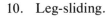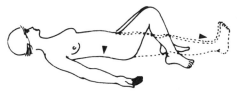

11. Diagonal curl-up.

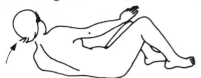

12. Relaxation on front when comfort permits.

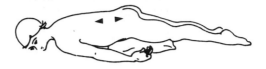

Phase V

Progressive abdominal exercises.

SUMMARY OF ESSENTIAL POSTPARTUM EXERCISES

Commence within 24 hours; repeat each exercise twice to start, progressing at your own pace through the phases. Relax and breathe deeply between each exercise. The sequence can be repeated in reverse order. Do the exercises at least twice daily.

Phase I

1. Deep breathing with abdominal wall tightening on outward breath.

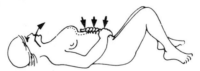

   2. Foot exercises. Bend, stretch, and rotate. Continue until walking around.

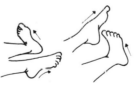

3. Stretch out the kinks.

4. Pelvic floor contractions.

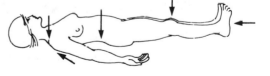

5. Pelvic-tilting.

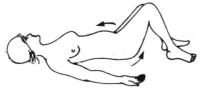

Before standing: Sit with legs over bed for a few minutes and swing the feet. Brace abdominals, buttocks, and pelvic floor when upright and walking around at first.

Posture check.

Relaxation: Lying on the front. Twice daily, at least half an hour.

Phase II

6. Leg-sliding.

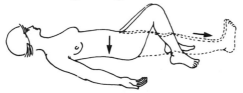

7. Bridging.

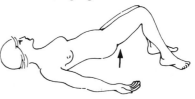

Phase III

Check for separation of the recti muscles after third day. Check stopping and starting of urine flow.

8. Straight curl-up.

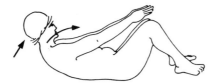

9. Diagonal curl-up.

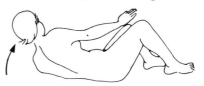

Phase IV

Progressive abdominal exercises.

SUMMARY OF ESSENTIAL PRENATAL EXERCISES

Do each exercise twice at first, progressing at your own pace to 5 times. The sequence can be repeated in reverse order. Relax and breathe deeply between each exercise.

1. Deep breathing with abdominal wall tightening on outward breath.

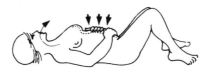

2. Foot exercises. Stretch, bend, and rotate.

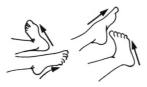

3. Stretch out the kinks. On the bed, against wall.

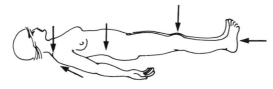

4. Pelvic floor contractions.
5. Pelvic-tilting: various positions (both pictures).

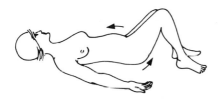
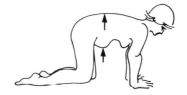

6. Leg-sliding.   7. Straight curl-up.

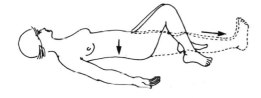
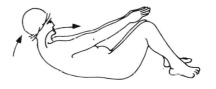

8. Bridging.   9. Diagonal curl-up.

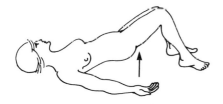
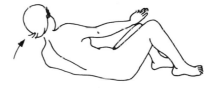

When standing: Roll over onto the knees and push arm with the arms. When rising from the floor, go on to one knee and straighten legs to stand.

Posture Check.

Relaxation: Twenty minutes' complete tension release in any position of comfort twice daily.

POSTURE CHECKLIST

Incorrect Posture   **To correct posture**

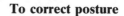

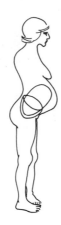 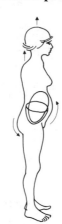

HEAD

If neck sags, chin pokes forward and whole body slumps.

Straighten neck, tuck chin in so body lines up.

SHOULDERS AND CHEST

Slouching cramps the rib cage and makes breathing difficult. Arms turn in.

Lift up through ribcage and pull back shoulder girdle. Roll arms out.

ABDOMEN AND BUTTOCKS

Slack muscles mean hollow back. Pelvis tilts forward.

Contract abdominals to flatten back. Tuck buttocks under and tilt pelvis back.

KNEES

Pressed back strains joints, pushes pelvis forward.

Bend to ease body weight over feet.

FEET

Weight on inner borders strains arches

Distribute body weight through center of each foot

Index